RESUSCITATION ASPECTS

Edited by **Theodoros Aslanidis**

Resuscitation Aspects
http://dx.doi.org/10.5772/66212
Edited by Theodoros Aslanidis

Contributors

Endre Zima, Enikő Kovács, Abbas Al Mutair, Carmen Diana Cimpoesu, Ovidiu Popa, Paul Nedelea, Daniel Molano-Franco, Maria Alejandra Velez Maya, Kirill Ivanov, Thais Russomano, Lucas Rehnberg, Javier Eslava-Schmalbach, Jose Ricardo Navarro Vargas, Shoa-Lin Lin, Hui-Chun Chen, Digna M Gonzalez-Otero, Marc Delaney, Bjorn Flora, Sahar Ahmad

Published by InTech

Janeza Trdine 9, 51000 Rijeka, Croatia

Publishing Process Manager Nina Kalinic
Technical Editor SPi Global
Cover InTech Design team

First published December, 2017
Printed in Croatia
Legal deposit, Croatia: National and University Library in Zagreb

Additional hard copies can be obtained from orders@intechopen.com

Resuscitation Aspects, Edited by Theodoros Aslanidis
p. cm.
Print ISBN 978-953-51-3663-7
Online ISBN 978-953-51-3664-4

For EU product safety concerns:
IN TECH d.o.o., Prolaz Marije Krucifikse Kozulić 3, 51000 Rijeka, Croatia,
info@intechopen.com or visit our website at intechopen.com.

Meet the editor

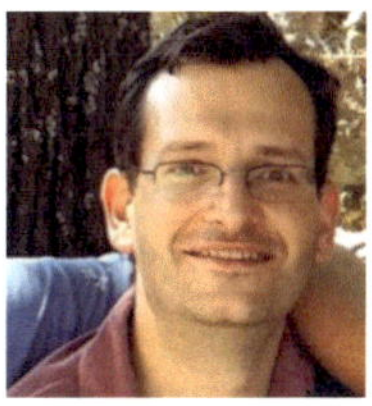

Dr. Theodoros K. Aslanidis received his Doctor of Medicine degree from Plovdiv Medical University, Bulgaria, in 2001. He served in the Hellenic Army Force as a medical doctor and then worked as a rural physician in Outhealth Centre, Iraklia and Serres' General Hospital, Greece. He moved to Thessaloniki where he completed his residency in anesthesiology in "Hippokratio" General Hospital, fellowship training at AHEPA University Hospital in Critical Care, and then a postgraduate program in Prehospital Emergency Medicine from the National Centre for Emergency Care. He serves as an editor in multiple medical journals. His research interests are medical writing, computational biostatistics, critical emergency medicine, and neuromonitoring. Dr. Aslanidis is currently working as Mobile Intensive Care Units' consultant at the National Centre of Emergency Care, Thessaloniki, Greece.

Contents

Preface

Resuscitation is a limitless field of clinical and basic science research and has led to great improvements in clinical care and outcomes over the past several decades. Over 50 years after the proposed "closed-chest cardiac massage" by Kouwenhoven, the challenge for better outcomes remains. The tremendous technological and medical advance only empowers our curiosity and impatience.

Today, we live in the era of transition from "classic" cardiopulmonary resuscitation (CPR) to something new. Everything that lies within the Advanced Life Support (ALS) protocols is under question. Assisted device CPR; alternative CPR position, e.g., prone CPR; patient-centric blood pressure–targeted CPR; and new training and feedback methods in resource-limited health systems are only some issues under research.

Within this frame, the present book, published by InTech®, highlights some interesting aspects of resuscitation. Divided into three sections, it passes from emphasizing details of resuscitation in special circumstances to possible future applications in the field.

The authors offer us not only a "vigorous" review of the current literature but also a research road path for further advancement—a road path that proves that resuscitation is anything but an exhausted subject for both the clinician and the researcher.

Dr. Theodoros Aslanidis
Hellenic National Center for Emergency Care,
Thessaloniki, Greece

Section 1

Introductory Issues

Chapter 1

The 10 Commandments of Resuscitation

Navarro-Vargas José Ricardo and
Eslava-Schmalbach Javier H.

Additional information is available at the end of the chapter

http://dx.doi.org/10.5772/intechopen.71729

Abstract

Cardiopulmonary cerebral resuscitation is a part of the theoretical and practical activities that must be mastered by health professionals who care for patients with haemodynamic compromise or cardiac arrest. Since Peter Safar, the father of western reanimatology, introduced the ABC-DEF-GHI mnemonic to help rescuers remember the steps of basic and advanced life support and postarrest management in a rapid, effective, and safe way, various mnemonic resources have been utilised to encode this knowledge in the long-term memory and help with fast retrieval. The purpose of this reflection article, based on different resuscitation workshops that have been carried out since 2000 at Colombian Society of Anaesthesiology and Resuscitation (S.C.A.R.E) and Universidad Nacional de Colombia., is to share a simple and practical set of 10 rules that must be followed in order to achieve successful resuscitation.

Keywords: cardiopulmonary resuscitation, cardiac arrest, sudden death, shock

1. Introduction

Cardiopulmonary cerebral resuscitation is critical among the competencies of every healthcare practitioner providing care to critically ill patients or patients who present with sudden haemodynamic decompensation or cardiorespiratory arrest.

Peter Safar, Austrian anaesthetist, three times nominated to the Nobel Prize in Medicine [1–4] for the wide scope of his scientific work focused on ensuring that "hearts and brains too young to die were resuscitated effectively," is considered the father of western reanimatology. He made significant contributions to the development of basic and advanced resuscitation with simple and sequential manoeuvres [1] and taught that resuscitation, an activity that must be performed in the midst of great stress, can be learnt with the purpose of not forgetting it and ensuring that a step-by-step procedure is followed. Also, at the end of the 1980s, the American cardiologist Richard Cummins [5, 6] introduced the chain of survival: a set of sequential and coordinated life-saving actions that have been validated by evidence over time. Convinced that success in any endeavour in life requires a good method, as well as a base of experience and favourable research outcomes like those obtained by defibrillation in the hands of the community [7], the authors wish to propose 10 simple, practical, and easy-to-remember rules to be considered during resuscitation.

2. The 10 commandments of resuscitation

2.1. First commandment: first the patient, then the monitor

Although technology has enabled great progress in refining control of the haemodynamic condition of the patients, there is no doubt about the importance of the semiology of the critically ill patient and the close surveillance on the part of the healthcare practitioner, considering that the patient is the original true source of information. Even in evidence-based medicine, the patient is one of the three fundamental pillars on which information is supported [8, 9].

It is not uncommon to find healthcare practitioners paying more attention to the parameters on the monitors than going to the patient as the primary source of information. This has given rise to medical errors in the diagnosis of "asystole" even before checking the patient (first 10 seconds in the first 10 minutes) [10, 11]; in the case of asystole, the worst possible diagnosis an individual can get, the protocol consists of confirming the effective placement of the electrodes, observing more than one lead, and increasing the amplitude of the electrocardiographic tracing.

2.2. Second commandment: check the pulse every 2 minutes

Consistent with the first commandment, cardiopulmonary resuscitation (CPR) cycles (compressions/ventilations) must occur at a constant rate of 30/2 (except in children, when two rescuers participate), and rescuers must switch and check pulse every 2 minutes [12]. However, in an editorial published in Resuscitation [13], Noordergraaf disagrees with the general algorithm of checking pulse every 2 minutes and attaches more importance to the type of arrest; if the aetiology is an H- or a T-like in pulseless electrical activity (PEA) and asystole, only 50% of patients have changed their condition to spontaneous circulation within 9 minutes, unlike what happens in shockable rhythms, which depend on electric therapy and require a discharge every 2 minutes. The objective of cardiopulmonary cerebral resuscitation is to help the heart resume circulation spontaneously with the least neurological compromise. If there is pulse there is life, hence the need to implement the 5th link in the chain of survival, which is the management of the "ischemia-reperfusion syndrome" or postcardiac arrest syndrome [14]. If there is a pulse, arterial pressure must be measured in order to determine the presence of vasodilation, characteristic of this syndrome. Hence, the need to be closely aware of these physiological changes is in order to initiate haemodynamic support infusions in a timely fashion.

2.3. Third commandment: if the rhythm changes, check the pulse!

The 2015 resuscitation guidelines emphasise prompt identification of the cardiac arrest as well as the quality of resuscitation. Chest compression frequency and depth are crucial for perfusion of the key organ, namely the brain [15]. Rhythm change is of the greatest importance in resuscitation because it indicates that the patient has either exhausted mitochondrial and cellular ATP reserves (going from VF to continuous asystole) or has gone into a rhythm with good prognosis. How is this determination made? The only way is the pulse: finding a pulse in a patient who was previously in cardiac arrest is one of the greatest achievements in resuscitation. If the patient is in exit rhythm, the next step is to treat postarrest syndrome, and if the cause of the arrest is identified, prognosis and recovery will be assured. There is increasingly more certainty regarding the fact that wide and slow complexes are of coronary aetiology, secondary to severe hyperkalemia or severe sodium channel blocker toxicity (these are agonal rhythms or that require urgent coronary intervention), unlike narrow fast rhythms, which are due to mechanical causes (cardiac tamponade, tension pneumothorax, pulmonary embolism) or hypovolemia [16]. The current use of point of care ultrasound (POCUS) has an excellent indication in the case of rhythm change with a pulse in order to rule out mechanical causes or hypovolemia as the factors leading to cardiac arrest [17].

If rhythm changes but does not recover, it is important to consider eight Hs and eight Ts among the possibilities for pulseless electrical activity [18]:

The eight Hs: hypoxia; hypovolemia; hyper-/hypokalemia; hydrogen ion (acidemia); hypothermia; hypoglycaemia; hyperthermia, malignant hypervagal.

The eight Ts: toxic (anaphylaxis/anaesthesia); tension pneumothorax; thrombosis/pulmonary embolism; thrombosis, coronary; tamponade, cardiac; trauma (haemorrhage, shock, cardiovascular injury); qT prolongation; pulmonary hypertension.

2.4. Fourth commandment: do not apply the algorithm in reverse. Wait-and-see management of exit arrhythmias

It is a serious mistake to consider the "exit" rhythm as the final heart rhythm because when the heart resumes circulation, it is in postischemic ventricular dysfunction or myocardial stunning [19].

Myocardial dysfunction takes time to recover and that is the reason why the "metabolic" phase of resuscitation requires critical management in the intensive care unit [20]. The sarcolemma is under calcium overload because the "ischemia-reperfusion" process injures the sarcoplasmic reticulum and alters calcium homeostasis; and there is enzymatic inactivation, lipid peroxidation, and mechanical actin/myosin coupling derangement due to collagen matrix injury [20, 21].

Regional flow may recover abruptly as a result of spontaneous cardiac circulation; however, regional muscle function recovery is insidious. The typical example of "myocardial stunning" happens when the infarcted heart is reperfused. On the other hand, the "hibernating" heart produces ventricular dysfunction before angioplasty or revascularisation, and regional myocardial function becomes normalised as soon as there is reperfusion [22]. In conclusion, pulse needs to be checked if there is a change of rhythm; and if there is a pulse, this rhythm (regardless of whether it is normal or arrhythmic) is called exit rhythm, and arterial pressure needs to be measured.

2.5. Fifth commandment: do not defibrillate a PEA or asystole rhythm

Successful defibrillation occurs when it suppresses a chaotic, disorganised, or very accelerated rhythm [as is the case in ventricular fibrillation (VF) or in pulseless ventricular tachycardia (PVT)] and places the heart in transient asystole so that it can restart with an organised rhythm. This may be achieved when there is sufficient ATP or else the heart goes into asystole and remains there because, without energy (prolonged arrest), it will not respond to electric discharge [23]. Regarding PEA, the arrest results from a special situation, which is not related to electrical instability leading to abnormal cardiac rhythm. Hs and Ts are good mnemonics to rule out probable causes of PEA/asystole, and management is not based on electric therapy but rather on solving the underlying cause of the arrest [24].

2.6. Sixth commandment: do not break the chain of survival

Across the years, the chain of survival has proven to be the key for the success of resuscitation, if all its steps are carried out carefully and in strict order. If there is a weak link, the chain will break. When Cummins et al. first published it [5], it consisted of four links: early access, early CPR, early defibrillation, early advanced care.

In 2010, the American Heart Association (AHA) added the fifth link that was missing in the chain, wherein lies the science and art of managing the "ischemia-reperfusion syndrome". Changes to the 2015 Guidelines included two distinct chains: the chain of survival for the patient who goes into cardiac arrest outside the hospital, which depends on the ability of the witnesses of the arrest to respond (first responders), and the chain for the inpatient whose survival will depend on an appropriate surveillance system for unstable patients (early diagnosis and warning/rapid response) and an organised advanced resuscitation system (Code Blue/Megacode) and teamwork [25].

2.7. Seventh commandment: in cardiac arrest, always apply three therapeutic options supported by level A evidence

Give compressions if there is cardiac arrest; give ventilations if there is respiratory arrest; defibrillate in case of ventricular fibrillation or PVT (**Figure 1**).

Of the 315 recommendations for changes to the 2015 Guidelines, only three had level A evidence (1%), which means that they were supported by controlled clinical trials or high quality meta-analyses, and only 78 (25%) were class I recommendations, meaning that the benefit is much higher than the risk (strong recommendation) [26].

2.8. Eighth commandment: do not give amiodarone in cases of tachycardia with *torsade de pointes* (twisting of the points)

Amiodarone is the versatile antiarrhythmic in resuscitation [27] because it acts on different cell channels. It is considered class I, II, III, and IV antiarrhythmic according to the Vaughan-Williams classification [28]. However, despite being an excellent antiarrhythmic in resuscitation, it also has arrhythmogenic effects, especially since it prolongs the QT interval and predisposes to helical polymorphic ventricular tachycardia or torsade. This form of arrhythmia produces haemodynamic instability that leads to cardiac arrest if it goes unrecognised and is

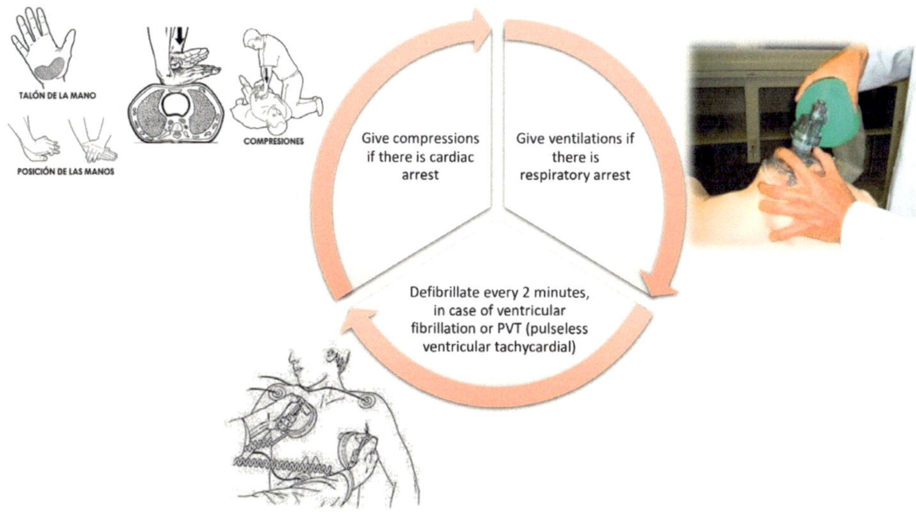

Figure 1. Therapeutic options with level A evidence. Note: PVT: pulseless ventricular tachycardia. Source: Author.

not treated on time, and among QT causes can be [29]: hypokalemia (normal levels: 3.5–5.3 mEq/L), hypomagnesemia (normal levels: 1.7–2.2 mg%), and antiarrhythmic toxicity.

2.9. Ninth commandment: give atropine only in case of symptomatic bradycardia

Severe bradyarrhythmias (produced by vagal responses during anaesthesia) respond to the use of atropine, an excellent parasympatholytic-anticholinergic agent that reduces vagal tone and increases sinus node frequency [25]. Atropine is a liposoluble tertiary amine of wide distribution in the body, which blocks muscarinic receptors. In cases of wide complex bradycardia, as is the case in high infra-His grade blocks, it has no effect because the block is below the AV node and it is actually contraindicated because atrial pacing may lead to cardiac arrest. Of these patients, 33% respond to transcutaneous pacemaker while waiting for assessment by the specialist and a definitive transvenous pacemaker [30, 31].

Atropine was excluded from cardiac arrest management (PEA-ASYSTOLE) already in the 2010 Guidelines; however, it must be kept in the crash cart because one of the Hs in the perioperative environment is "hypervagal response" [32].

2.10. Tenth commandment: assertive communication and clear messages

It has been estimated that 400,000 patients die every year because of medical errors, and 80% of these are attributed to communication errors and failures in nontechnical skills [33].

There is still a failure on the part of residents to adhere to the use of checklists, which have resulted in great progress in the control of adverse events [34].

Advanced life support teams (Code Blue/Megacode) must be characterised by excellent communication and leadership, which among nontechnical skills, are key to resuscitation success.

3. Conclusion

Cardiopulmonary cerebral resuscitation is a healthcare activity that requires an orderly step-by-step use of manoeuvres, and technical and nontechnical skills, where adherence to 10 rules described here reinforces the strength of all the links in the chain of survival and ensures a responsible, judicious, and effective job.

Author details

Navarro-Vargas José Ricardo[1,2,3]* and Eslava-Schmalbach Javier H.[1,2,3]

*Address all correspondence to: jrnavarrov@unal.edu.co

1 Hospital Universitario Nacional de Colombia, Bogotá, Colombia

2 Sociedad Colombiana de Anestesiología y Reanimación (S.C.A.R.E.), Confederación Latinoamericana de Sociedades de Anestesiología (CLASA), Bogotá, Colombia

3 Facultad de Medicina, Universidad Nacional de Colombia, Bogotá, Colombia

References

[1] Grenvik A, Kochanek PM. The incredible career of Peter J. Safar, MD: The Michelangelo of acute medicine. Critical Care Medicine. 2004;**32**(2 Suppl):S3-S7

[2] Kochanek PM, Grenvik A. A tribute to Peter J. Safar, MD. Critical Care Medicine. 2003; **31**(11):2571-2573

[3] Mitka M, Peter J. Safar, MD. "Father of CPR", innovator, teacher, humanist. Journal of the American Medical Association 2003;**289**(19):2485–2486

[4] Safar P. On the future of reanimatology. Academic Emergency Medicine. 2000;**7**(1):75-89

[5] Cummins RO, Ornato JP, Thies WH, Pepe PE. Improving survival from sudden cardiac arrest: The "chain of survival" concept. A statement for health professionals from the advanced cardiac life support subcommittee and the emergency cardiac care committee, American Heart Association. Circulation. 1991;**83**(5):1832-1847

[6] Navarro-Vargas J. Temas selectos de reanimación cerebro cardiopulmonar (RCCP) (e-book). Bogota: Universidad Nacional de Colombia; Sociedad Colombiana de Anestesiologia y Reanimación (S.C.A.R.E.); 2015. Available from: https://www.amazon.com/Temas-selectos-reanimaci%C3%B3n-Cerebro-cardiopulmonar-Spanish-ebook/dp/B01567D46S

[7] Navarro-Vargas J, Muñoz-Corena R. Historia de la terapia eléctrica en reanimación. Revista Cubana de Anestesiología [Internet]. 2017 18 Julio 2017;**16**(1). Available from: http://bvs.sld.cu/revistas/scar/vol16_1_17/scarsu117.htm

[8] Lazar E. What Is Evidence-Based Practice and why Is it Important? 2015. Available from: https://www.functionalmovement.com/articles/651/what_is_evidence-based_practice_and_why_is_it_important

[9] Navarro-Vargas J, Eslava-Schmalbach J, Cruz L. Semiología del paciente crítico ¿La clínica y la monitoria invasiva ¿Son excluyentes o se complementan? Bogota: Sociedad Cundinamarquesa de Anestesiologia; 2009

[10] Eberle B, Dick WF, Schneider T, Wisser G, Doetsch S, Tzanova I. Checking the carotid pulse check: Diagnostic accuracy of first responders in patients with and without a pulse. Resuscitation. 1996;**33**(2):107-116

[11] Ramanathan G, Kumar JM, Sivarajan G, Umadevi P. Is flat line truly asystole? Indian Journal of Anaesthesia. 2015;**59**(8):528-529

[12] Harsoor SS. Cardio pulmonary resuscitation 2010 – improve the quality of care. Indian Journal of Anaesthesia. 2010;**54**(2):91-94

[13] Noordergraaf GJ, Noordergraaf A. What should determine loop time during CPR: A generic algorithm or the patient's initial rhythm? Resuscitation. 2014;**85**(1):9-10

[14] Navarro-Vargas J, Díaz J. Sindrome posparo cardiaco. Revista Colombiana de Anestesiología. 2014;**42**:107-113

[15] Neumar RW, Shuster M, Callaway CW, Gent LM, Atkins DL, Bhanji F, et al. Part 1: Executive summary: 2015 American Heart Association guidelines update for cardiopulmonary resuscitation and emergency cardiovascular care. Circulation. 2015;**132**(18 Suppl 2): S315-S367

[16] Mehta C, Brady W. Pulseless electrical activity in cardiac arrest: Electrocardiographic presentations and management considerations based on the electrocardiogram. The American Journal of Emergency Medicine. 2012;**30**(1):236-239

[17] Littmann L, Bustin DJ, Haley MW. A simplified and structured teaching tool for the evaluation and management of pulseless electrical activity. Medical Principles and Practice. 2014;**23**(1):1-6

[18] Moitra VK, Gabrielli A, Maccioli GA, O'Connor MF. Anesthesia advanced circulatory life support. Canadian Journal of Anaesthesia. 2012;**59**(6):586-603

[19] Bolli R. Mechanism of myocardial "stunning". Circulation. 1990;**82**(3):723-738

[20] Weisfeldt ML, Becker LB. Resuscitation after cardiac arrest: A 3-phase time-sensitive model. Journal of the American Medical Association. 2002;**288**(23):3035-3038

[21] Canty JM Jr., Suzuki G Myocardial perfusion and contraction in acute ischemia and chronic ischemic heart disease. Journal of Molecular and Cellular Cardiology 2012;**52**(4):822–831

[22] Conti CR. The stunned and hibernating myocardium: A brief review. Clinical Cardiology. 1991;**14**(9):708-712

[23] Kleinman ME, Brennan EE, Goldberger ZD, Swor RA, Terry M, Bobrow BJ, et al. Part 5: Adult basic life support and cardiopulmonary resuscitation quality: 2015 American Heart Association guidelines update for cardiopulmonary resuscitation and emergency cardiovascular care. Circulation. 2015;**132**(18 Suppl 2):S414-S435

[24] Lavonas EJ, Drennan IR, Gabrielli A, Heffner AC, Hoyte CO, Orkin AM, et al. Part 10: Special circumstances of resuscitation: 2015 American Heart Association guidelines update for cardiopulmonary resuscitation and emergency cardiovascular care. Circulation. 2015;**132**(18 Suppl 2):S501-S518

[25] American Heart Association. Highlights of the 2015 American Heart Association. Guidelines Update for CPR and ECC2015 19 Julio 2017. Available from: http://eccguidelines.heart.org/wp-content/uploads/2015/10/2015-AHA-Guidelines-Highlights-English.pdf

[26] Morrison LJ, Gent LM, Lang E, Nunnally ME, Parker MJ, Callaway CW, et al. Part 2: Evidence evaluation and Management of Conflicts of interest: 2015 American Heart Association guidelines update for cardiopulmonary resuscitation and emergency cardiovascular care. Circulation. 2015;**132**(18 Suppl 2):S368-S382

[27] Comité de Reanimación, Sociedad Colombiana de Anestesiología y Reanimación. Medicamentos en reanimación. Soporte vital avanzado, Guía 2015. Bogota: Sociedad Colombiana de Anestesiologia y Reanimación, S.C.A.R.E.; 2015

[28] Gonzalez ER, Kannewurf BS, Ornato JP. Intravenous amiodarone for ventricular arrhythmias: overview and clinical use. Resuscitation. 1998;**39**(1-2):33-42

[29] Ayad RF, Assar MD, Simpson L, Garner JB, Schussler JM. Causes and management of drug-induced long QT syndrome. Proceedings (Baylor University Medical Center). 2010; **23**(3):250-255

[30] Laverde C. Paro cardiaco durante colecistectomía laparoscópica. Revista Colombiana de Anestesiología. 2013;**41**(4):298-301

[31] Levis JT. ECG diagnosis: Complete heart block. The Permanente Journal. 2011;**15**(2):90

[32] Dos Reis F, Ferez D, Gomes do Amaral J. Actualización de las directrices de resucitación cardiopulmonar de interés del anestesista. Revista Brasileira de Anestesiologia 2011;**61**(5):341–350

[33] James JT. A new, evidence-based estimate of patient harms associated with hospital care. Journal of Patient Safety. 2013;**9**(3):122-128

[34] Heck MC, Huges P, Konia M. An evaluation of CA-1 Residents' adherence to a standardized handoff checklist. The Journal of Education in Perioperative Medicine. 2017;**19**(1): E502

Section 2

Special Issues

Chapter 2

Cardiopulmonary Resuscitation in Special Circumstances

Diana Carmen Cimpoesu and Tudor Ovidiu Popa

Additional information is available at the end of the chapter

http://dx.doi.org/10.5772/intechopen.70304

Abstract

Cardiopulmonary resuscitation (CPR) in special circumstances includes the emergency intervention for special causes, special environments and special patients. Special causes cover the potential reversible causes of cardiac arrest that must be identified or excluded during any resuscitation, divided into two groups, 4Hs and 4Ts: hypoxia, hypo-/hyperkalaemia and other electrolyte disorders, hypo-/hyperthermia, hypervolemia, tension pneumothorax, tamponade (cardiac), thrombosis (coronary or pulmonary) and toxins. The special environments section includes recommendations for the treatment of cardiac arrest occurring in specific locations: cardiac surgery, catheterisation laboratory, dialysis unit, dental surgery, commercial airplanes or air ambulances, field of play, difficult environment (e.g. drowning, high altitude, avalanche and electrical injuries) or mass casualty incident. CPR for special patients gives guidance for the patients with severe comorbidities (asthma, heart failure with ventricular assist devices, neurological disease and obesity) and pregnancy women or elderly people.

Keywords: cardiopulmonary resuscitation, special causes, special patients, special environment

1. Introduction

According to the actual guidelines for cardiopulmonary resuscitation (CPR), early recognition and calling for help, early defibrillation, high-quality resuscitation with minimal interruption of chest compressions and treatment of reversible causes are the most important interventions that can improve the outcomes after cardiac arrest [1–4].

The 2015 Guidelines for resuscitation published by European Resuscitation Council divide the resuscitation in special circumstances into three parts: special causes, special environments and special patients [4].

The first part covers treatment of potentially reversible causes of cardiac arrest, for which specific treatment exists and which are divided into two groups of four, called 'the 4Hs and 4Ts': hypoxia; hypo-/hyperkalaemia and other electrolyte disorders; hypo-/hyperthermia; hypovolaemia; tension pneumothorax; tamponade (cardiac tamponade); thrombosis (coronary and pulmonary) and toxins (poisoning) [1, 4].

The second part covers cardiac arrest in special environments, where universal guidelines should be modified due to specific locations or location-specific causes of cardiac arrest [1, 5].

The third part contains the recommendation for the patients with specific conditions and those with certain long-term comorbidities, where a modified approach and different treatment decisions may be necessary [4].

2. Special causes

Hypoxia is usually a consequence of asphyxia, which is defined as pathological changes caused by lack of oxygen in respired air, resulting in a deficiency of oxygen in the blood (hypoxia) and an increase in carbon dioxide in the blood and tissues (hypercapnia). Symptoms usually include irregular and disturbed respirations, or a complete absence of breathing, and pallor or cyanosis. Asphyxia may occur whenever there is an interruption in the normal exchange of oxygen and carbon dioxide between the lungs and the outside air. Some common causes are drowning, electric shock, hanging, suffocation, lodging of a foreign body in the air passages, inhalation of smoke and poisonous gases, and trauma to or disease of the lungs or air passages. Hypoxia requires ventilation with airway adjuncts that need to be verified to be placed correctly. There is necessary to check breath sounds at regular time intervals to ensure that the endotracheal tube has not slipped out of the trachea or to identify the presence of pneumothorax. Also is necessary to verify the source of oxygen (an oxygen cylinder or the piped oxygen supply).

The effective ventilation with supplementary oxygen during the early moment of resuscitation is essential during CPR. Also, it is recommended to monitor the efficacy of ventilation via capnometry which measures end-tidal CO_2. CPR is indicated to monitor the effectiveness of manoeuvres by obtaining a value between 10 and 20 mmHg. An abrupt increase of end-tidal CO_2 values indicates return of spontaneous circulation (ROSC). If after oro-tracheal intubation, there is no waveform during CPR, but a flat line, this should alert for misplacement of endotracheal tube [1, 4, 6].

Electrolyte abnormalities can cause cardiac arrhythmias or cardiac arrest. Life-threatening arrhythmias are most commonly associated with potassium disorders. The main causes of hyperkalaemia are renal failure, drugs (e.g. angiotensin-converting enzyme inhibitors, angiotensin II receptor antagonists, potassium-sparing diuretics), rhabdomyolysis, metabolic acidosis, Addison's disease, diet. The treatment strategies for hyperkalaemia are cardiac protection, shifting potassium into cells, removing potassium from the body, monitoring serum potassium and blood glucose [1, 4, 6].

Hypothermia: accidental hypothermia is defined as an involuntary decrease of body core temperature <35°C. It is divided in five stages according to central core temperature: 1. mild hypothermia (conscious, shivering, core temperature 35–32°C); 2. moderate hypothermia (impaired consciousness without shivering, core temperature 32–28°C); 3. severe hypothermia (unconscious, vital signs present, core temperature 28–24°C); 4. cardiac arrest or low flow state (no or minimal vital signs, core temperature <24°C) and 5. death due to irreversible hypothermia (core temperature <13.7°C) [4].

Hypothermia decreases oxygen consumption at cellular level, so the heart and the brain can tolerate for a longer period of time cardiac arrest. This is the basic concept of the protective effect of hypothermia in cardiac arrest. Sometimes complete neurological recovery can be found even after prolonged cardiac arrest, but only if hypothermia was installed before respiratory arrest [1, 4, 6–9].

The first measure is to remove the patient from cold environment, remove clothes which are usually wet or cold and try to prevent any other heat loss. Quick mobilisation of patient with hypothermia can induce arrhythmias [1, 4, 6].

Hypothermia need to be treated with gradual rewarming using normal or electric blankets and warm IV fluids. The goal is to achieve an increase of temperature with a rate of 1–1.5°C per hour. It should be used IV fluid (normal saline, for example) heated at approx. 40°C and also gastric lavage, peritoneal lavage, bladder lavage, using fluids heated at approx. 40°C.

Monitor electrolytes disorder hourly, especially hyperkalaemia, which can appear during heating manoeuvres. Oxygen should be delivered also heated and humidified at 40°C, using a mechanical ventilator, after oro-tracheal intubation [1, 4–6].

Regarding CPR manoeuvres, in case of hypothermia-associated thoracic stiffness is present. Thus, chest compressions are harder to perform, and ventilation will require higher pressures than in normal situation [1, 4, 5, 7–9].

In case of ROSC, pulse in patients with hypothermia is very weak due to peripheral vasoconstriction, so is needed to consider Doppler examination to assess correctly the presence or absence of circulation.

Hypothermic patients without signs of cardiac instability (systolic blood pressure ≥90 mmHg, absence of ventricular arrhythmias or core temperature ≥28°C) can be rewarmed externally using minimally invasive techniques (warm air and warm intravenous fluid). Patients with signs of cardiac instability should be resuscitated in the field and transferred directly to a centre capable of extracorporeal life support (ECLS) [1, 4–9].

Hypovolaemia is a potentially treatable cause of cardiac arrest that usually results from a haemorrhage, but relative hypovolaemia may also occur in patients with severe vasodilation (e.g. anaphylaxis, sepsis). In case of anaphylaxis with relative hypovolaemia, the immediate treatment with intramuscular adrenaline is the treatment of choice, followed by IV fluids and corticoids prolonged CPR may be necessary [1, 4, 6, 10].

History of fluid or blood loss may be available. Rectal examination can identify massive lower GI bleeding; nasogastric intubation can identify massive upper GI bleeding, and bedside FAST can diagnose massive intraperitoneal bleeding. Treatment is with fluids (crystalloids, colloids), administered rapidly IV and blood products. If colloids are administered, blood samples are necessary before of this, to work compatibility cross-match blood test, because colloids can interfere with the results [1, 4, 6].

Tension pneumothorax: the mortality from traumatic cardiac arrest (TCA) is very high. The most common cause of death is haemorrhage, but the patients with trauma could have other reversible causes: hypoxia, tension pneumothorax, cardiac tamponade, and all of them must be immediately treated [1, 4, 5, 11–14].

The new treatment algorithm for traumatic cardiac arrest was developed to prioritise the sequence of life-saving measures. Chest compressions should not delay the treatment of reversible causes.

Suspect of tension pneumothorax during cardiac resuscitation if breath sounds are unequal on chest auscultation after verifying correct endotracheal tube placement. Other useful clinical sign for diagnosis are one immobile, distended hemi thorax; hyper resonance with percussion over the chest wall; trachea deviation to opposite side of tension pneumothorax and jugular veins distention. Treatment is immediate needle decompression or other technique to decompress the chest in TCA—to perform unilateral or bilateral thoracotomies in the 4th intercostal space. In the presence of positive pressure ventilation, thoracotomies are likely to be more effective than needle thoracentesis and quicker than inserting a chest tube [1, 5, 11–14].

Cardiac tamponade is the underlying cause of approximately 10% of cardiac arrest in trauma. Whereas there are TCA and penetrating trauma to the chest or epigastrium, immediate resuscitative thoracotomy (RT) can be lifesaving. If thoracotomy is not possible, consider ultrasound guided pericardiocentesis to treat cardiac arrest with cardiac tamponade. Cardiac tamponade is best identified during resuscitation by bedside transthoracic ultrasound. This requires brief interruption of chest compressions up to 10 s. Another useful ECG sign in cardiac tamponade is represented by microvoltage, in traumatic event context. Treatment of tamponade causing cardiac arrest is bedside pericardiocentesis [1, 4, 5, 12–14].

Thrombosis for the patients with out-of-hospital cardiac arrest (OHCA) of suspected cardiac origin, the transfer to the hospital with continuing CPR could be a solution in case of acute coronary syndrome–coronary thrombosis. Ground transport may be beneficial in selected patients where there is immediate hospital access to the catheterisation laboratory and an infrastructure providing prehospital and in-hospital teams experienced in mechanical or haemodynamic support and percutaneous coronary intervention (PCI) with ongoing CPR [1, 4, 15–19].

Acute coronary thrombosis or acute myocardial infarction is one of the most common causes of cardiac arrest. Risk factors are a history of coronary artery disease and initial rhythm of VF/VT. Cardiac catheterisation after resuscitation is an underused procedure. A 12-lead ECG in the immediate postcardiac arrest state can identify an ST-elevation acute myocardial infarction and allows for arrangements of immediate coronary angiography. Myocardial and neurologic function can improve after percutaneous coronary intervention following cardiac arrest. Therefore, after ROSC, especially in the face of post-ROSC, ECG evidence of acute myocardial infarction, cardiac catheterisation and percutaneous coronary revascularisation is recommended, if available and appropriate [1, 4, 5].

Acute pulmonary embolism will be suspected by clinical symptoms such as dyspnoea, chest pain and syncope, either only one of this or in combination. Most frequent patient-related predisposing factors for developing pulmonary embolism include age, history of previous deep vein thrombosis, active cancer, neurological disease with extremity paresis, medical condition causing prolonged bed rest, such as heart or acute respiratory failure or post-surgery, congenital or acquired thrombophilia, hormone replacement therapy and oral contraceptive therapy [1, 4, 5, 15–17].

Electrocardiographic signs of RV strain, such as inversion of T waves in leads V1–V4, a QR pattern in lead V1, the classic pattern of S1Q3T3 ECG type and incomplete or complete right bundle-branch block, may be helpful also to raise the suspicion for pulmonary embolism.

The administration of fibrinolytic when pulmonary embolism is the suspected cause of cardiac arrest remains the actual recommendation. Pulmonary embolism causing cardiac arrest requires fibrinolysis or embolectomy. However, the diagnosis is rarely made at time of collapse, and even then, most systems are not geared to make such prompt diagnosis and initiate the necessary procedures for embolectomy [1, 4, 5, 15, 16, 19].

Fibrinolytic agents could be considered during cardiac arrest from suspected pulmonary embolism on a case-by-case basis. Factors suggestive of pulmonary embolism causing cardiac arrest include two of three signs/symptoms (prearrest respiratory distress, altered mental status or shock); arrest witnessed by a physician or emergency medical technician and PEA as the first or primary arrest rhythm. Ongoing CPR is not a contraindication to fibrinolysis, and after fibrinolytic drug is administered, CPR should be continued for at least 60–90 min before terminating resuscitation attempts [1, 4, 15–18, 20].

Toxics: airway obstruction and respiratory arrest secondary to a decreased conscious level is a common cause of cardiac arrest after accidental or self-poisoning. There are few specific therapeutic measures for poisoning that are useful immediately and during cardiopulmonary resuscitation and improve outcomes: decontamination, enhancing elimination and the use of specific antidotes.

The preferred method of gastrointestinal decontamination in patients with protected airways is activated charcoal but is most effective only if given within first hour from ingestion. Drug overdose is rarely identified as a cause of cardiac arrest during the resuscitation process. In the event of antidepressant overdose, administer IV sodium bicarbonate. Lipid emulsion infusion may be useful in cardiac arrest associated with cyclic antidepressants or local anaesthetics.

Opioid poisoning causes respiratory depression followed by respiratory insufficiency or respiratory arrest. The use of naloxone can prevent the need for intubation. The initial doses of naloxone are 0.4–2 mg IV, IO, IM or SC and may be repeated every 2–3 min. Additional doses may be needed every 20–60 min. Titrate the dose until the victim is breathing adequately and has protective airway reflexes [4, 5, 21].

3. Special environment

The special environments include cardiac arrest in specific locations: operating theatre, cardiac surgery, catheterisation laboratory, dialysis unit, dental surgery, commercial airplanes or medical helicopters, field of play, outside environment (e.g. drowning, remote area, high altitude, avalanche, lightning strike and electrical injuries) or the scene of a mass casualty incident.

Cardiac arrest following major **cardiac surgery** is relatively common in the immediate postoperative phase. Perioperative cardiac arrest may be caused by the physiological effects of the surgery, bleeding, general anaesthesia (failure of ventilation, medication-related events, complications associated with central venous access, drugs or blood administration, perioperative myocardial infarction) [22–24] or complications relating to pre-existing comorbidities.

The management of perioperative cardiac arrest starts with advanced life support (ALS) algorithm, but with appropriate modifications depending on the cause identified. Key to successful resuscitation is recognition of the need to perform emergency re-sternotomy, especially in the context of tamponade or haemorrhage, where external chest compressions may be ineffective. Re-sternotomy should be performed within 5 min if other interventions have failed.

Cardiac arrest may occur during percutaneous coronary intervention (PCI) for ST-elevation myocardial infarction (STEMI) or non-STEMI, or it may be a complication during angiography as air or thrombus embolism in the coronary artery, artery intima dissection or pericardial tamponade. A defibrillator must be available in the angiography room, and self-adhesive defibrillation pads may already be placed at the beginning of the procedure in high-risk patients.

Cardiac arrest from shockable rhythms (ventricular fibrillation or pulseless ventricular tachycardia) during **cardiac catheterisation** should immediately be treated with up to three stacked shocks before starting chest compressions. Use of mechanical chest compression devices during angiography is recommended to ensure high-quality chest compressions and reduce the radiation of the personnel during angiography with ongoing CPR.

Most of the standard reversible causes (4Hs and 4Ts) apply to **dialysis patients**. Electrolyte disorders, particularly hyperkalaemia and hypoxia, due to fluid overload with pulmonary edema are most common causes of cardiac arrest in dialysis unit.

During cardiopulmonary resuscitation, it follows the universal ALS algorithm, and the dialysis access open for drug administration A shockable rhythm (VF/pulseless VT) is more common in patients undergoing haemodialysis than in the general population [25–29]. So the delay in delivering defibrillation must be minimised.

In **dental surgery**, causes of cardiac arrest are related to pre-existing comorbidities (acute myocardial infarction, grand mal seizures or exacerbation of asthma), loss of airway patency related to the primary pathology or complications of the procedure (e.g. bleeding, secretions, tissue swelling) or anaphylaxis to local anaesthetics.

The patient will not be moved from the dental chair to start CPR, the dental chair will be reclined into a horizontal position or a stool will be placed under the head to increase its stability during CPR. Consider the over-the-head technique of CPR, if access of the chest is limited [30–32].

Cardiopulmonary resuscitation on the airplane: in case of cardiac arrest, universal algorithm for adult basic life support and automated external defibrillation (AED) will be followed, but performance of CPR is limited in an aircraft due to space restriction, so consider the transfer of the patient to a larger space. Consider an over-the-head technique of CPR if access precludes conventional PR [30–32].

If the CPR equipment is available, attach oxygen to the facemask or self-inflating bag. Request immediate flight diversion to the nearest appropriate airport. The in-flight use of AEDs aboard commercial airplanes can result in up to 50% survival to hospital discharge [4]. AEDs and appropriate CPR equipment should be mandatory on board of all commercial aircraft in Europe, including regional and low-cost carriers [33].

The incidence of cardiac arrest on board of **helicopter emergency medical services** (HEMS) and air ambulances is low. Cardiac arrest may occur in-flight, both in patients being transported from a primary intervention site and also critical patients transferred between hospital [34]. The pre-flight preparation is important for the patients with high risk of cardiac arrest and use of mechanical chest compression devices are emphasised [4, 5].

Sudden and unexpected collapse of a sportsman **during exercises or on the field of play** is likely to be cardiac in origin and requires rapid recognition, initiating basic life support (BLS) and early defibrillation. If the athlete responds to resuscitation, then he/she must be transported immediately to the nearest cardiac centre for further evaluation and treatment [4, 5].

For **drowning patients**, bystanders play an essential role in early rescue and high-quality resuscitation. The victim needs to be removed from the water promptly. Resuscitation strategies for those in respiratory or cardiac arrest continue to prioritise oxygenation and ventilation. Inflation should take about 1 s and be sufficient to see the chest rise [4, 5].

Rescue breaths/ventilation will continue until an ALS team arrives and is ready to intubate the victim. Palpation of the pulse is not always reliable. As soon as possible, use information from monitoring modalities such as the ECG, end-tidal CO_2, and echocardiography to confirm the diagnosis of cardiac arrest. If the drowning victim is hypothermic or hypovolaemic, modify the ALS approach in accordance with the treatment of hypothermia and give IV warm fluid.

The chances of good outcome from cardiac arrest in **difficult terrain or mountains** may be reduced because of delayed access and prolonged transport. There is a recognised role of air rescue and availability of AEDs in remote but often-visited locations [4, 35]. Resuscitation at high altitude does not differ from standard CPR. CPR is more exhausting for a single rescuer than at sea level, due to lower pO_2, and the average number of effective chest compressions may decrease within the first minute [36].

For **avalanche victims** in cardiac arrest, prolonged CPR and extracorporeal rewarming are indicated. Cardiac arrest secondary to avalanche is mainly due to asphyxia associated with trauma and hypothermia. In all cases, extricate the body gently and use spinal precautions. Extracorporeal life support (ECLS) is indicated if the duration of burial is >60 min, core temperature at extrication is <30°C and serum potassium at hospital admission is ≤8 mmol L^{-1} [4, 35, 37].

Safety measures are essential for providing CPR to the victim of an **electrical injury** [4]. Factors influencing the severity of electrical injury include the current type alternating (AC) or direct (DC), voltage, magnitude of energy delivered, resistance to current flow, the area and duration of contact. As with industrial and domestic electric shock, after lightning strikes death is caused by cardiac or respiratory arrest [38–41].

Ensure that any power source is switched off and approach the casualty only if it is safe and start standard BLS and ALS without delay. Airway management may be difficult, and early tracheal intubation is needed if there are electrical burns around the face and neck. Head and spine trauma can occur after electrocution, and the spine immobilisation must be performed.

VF is the commonest initial arrhythmia after high-voltage AC shock, and prompt defibrillation is essential. Asystole is more common after DC shock with standard ALS protocols.

Unlike normal circumstances, CPR is not usually initiated in **mass casualty incidents** (MCI), in order to avoid delaying potentially effective treatment for the critically ill but salvageable victims. This critical decision depends on available medical and paramedical resources in relation to the number of casualties.

A triage system should be used to prioritise treatment and, if the number of casualties overwhelms the prehospital medical resources, withhold CPR for the patients without signs of life [1, 5]. For triage, the START triage is used. The first step is that everyone able to walk is directed to clear the scene, and respiratory status of nonwalking patients is assessed. If the casualty does not breathe, open the airway using head tilt and chin lift or jaw thrust. Assess breathing for no more than 10 s and if a patient does not begin breathing is declared dead. If an unresponsive victim is breathing normally, turn them into the recovery position and label as red-highest priority for treatment. The same goes for the patient with sign of hemodynamic instability.

> Perform life-saving interventions in patients triaged as red (highest priority) to prevent cardiac arrest: control major haemorrhage, open airway using basic techniques, perform chest decompression for tension pneumothorax, use antidotes and consider initial rescue breaths in a nonbreathing child [42].

4. Special patients

Special patients with special guidance for CPR are considered to be the patients with severe comorbidities: asthma, heart failure with ventricular assist devices, neurological disease, obesity and those with specific physiological conditions (pregnancy, elderly people).

Cardiac arrest in a patient with **asthma** is often a terminal event after a hypoxemic period or it may be sudden. CA is linked to:

- severe bronchospasm and mucous plugging leading to asphyxia;
- cardiac arrhythmias caused by hypoxia, by stimulant drugs (beta-adrenergic agonists, aminophylline) or electrolyte abnormalities;
- dynamic hyperinflation, that is, auto positive end-expiratory pressure (auto-PEEP), can occur in mechanically ventilated asthmatics. Gradual build-up of pressure occurs and reduces venous return and blood pressure and determines heart failure;
- tension pneumothorax uni/bilateral.

These high-risk patients should be treated to prevent deterioration with oxygen to achieve an SpO_2 94–98%, inhaled beta-2 agonists (salbutamol 5 mg) or intravenous beta-2 agonists for those patients in whom inhaled therapy cannot be used reliably, nebulised anticholinergics (ipratropium, 0.5 mg 4–6 hourly), nebulised magnesium sulphate, intravenous corticosteroids, intravenous bronchodilators and aminophylline, a dose of 5 mg kg^{-1} over 20–30 min. In cases of severe asthma associated with dehydration and hypovolemia IV fluids are necessary.

In case of cardiac arrest BLS is performed according to standard guidelines. Ventilation could be difficult because of increased airway resistance.

Modifications to standard ALS guidelines include the need for early tracheal intubation. The peak airway pressures recorded during ventilation of patients with severe asthma are significantly higher than the normal lower oesophageal sphincter pressure (approximately 20 cm H_2O) [43, 44].

Respiratory rates of 8–10 breaths/min and a tidal volume required for a normal chest rise during CPR should minimise dynamic hyperinflation of the lungs [air trapping].

Tidal volume depends on inspiratory time and inspiratory flow. Lung emptying depends on expiratory time and expiratory flow. In mechanically ventilated severe asthmatics, increasing the expiratory time (achieved by reducing the respiratory rate) provides only moderate gains in terms of reduced gas trapping when a minute volume of less than 10 L min^{-1} is used [44].

Dynamic hyperinflation increases transthoracic impedance [45] but modern impedance-compensated biphasic defibrillation waveforms are no less effective in patients with higher impedance. Consider increasing defibrillation energy if the first shock is unsuccessful, and a manual defibrillator is available [4].

There is no good evidence for the use of open-chest cardiac compressions in patients with asthma-associated cardiac arrest. Looking through the four H's and four T's will identify potentially reversible causes of asthma-related cardiac arrest, often tension pneumothorax. This pathologic situation may be indicated by unilateral expansion of the chest wall, shifting of the trachea and subcutaneous emphysema. If a pneumothorax is suspected, perform needle decompression using a large-gauge cannula, followed by insertion of a chest tube.

In patients with **ventricular assist devices** (VADs), confirmation of cardiac arrest may be difficult. The management of patients with VADs is more complex, in that a cardiac arrest may be due to mechanical failure and may be actions specific to the device that are required. In any cases, external chest compression in patients with ventricular assist devices is not successful without damage to the VAD.

Transthoracic/transesophageal echocardiography, capnography or Doppler flow in a major artery may assist in the cardiac arrest diagnosis. If cardiac arrest is confirmed, start CPR, check the rhythm and perform defibrillation for shockable rhythms (VF/VT), start pacing for asystole. If during the first 10 days of surgery, cardiac arrest does not respond to defibrillation, perform re-sternotomy immediately.

Cardiac arrest associated with **acute neurological disease** is relatively uncommon and can appear in subarachnoid haemorrhage, intracerebral haemorrhage, epileptic seizures and ischemic stroke and in brain injury associated with trauma [46].

The mechanism of cardiac arrest in neurological disease is related to:

(a) loss of consciousness, causing airway obstruction, hypoxemia and respiratory arrest followed by cardiac arrest, or an increased risk of aspiration of gastric contents into the lungs

(b) respiratory and cardiac depression caused by compression of the brain stem

(c) arrhythmias and myocardial dysfunction associated with acute neurological injury (e.g. sub-arachnoid haemorrhage)

(d) Sudden unexpected death in epilepsy [4].

Patients with subarachnoid haemorrhage may have ECG changes that suggest an acute coronary syndrome. Whether a computed tomography brain scan is done before or after coronary angiography will depend on clinical judgement regarding the likelihood of a subarachnoid haemorrhage versus acute coronary syndrome.

For resuscitation of **obese patients**, in order to maintain sufficient depth of chest compressions (approximately 5 cm but no more than 6 cm), consider changing rescuers more frequently than the standard 2-min interval. Early tracheal intubation by an experienced physician is recommended. Use of mechanical resuscitation devices is limited by the slope of the anterior chest wall and thoracic dimensions.

Optimal defibrillation energy levels in obese patients are unknown [4]. So the recommended energy remains the same (150–360 J). Unlike monophasic defibrillators, modern biphasic defibrillators are impedance compensated and adjust their output according to the patient's impedance. Defibrillation protocols for obese patients should therefore follow those recommended for patients with a normal BMI and consider higher shock energies for defibrillation if initial defibrillation attempts fail.

For the **pregnant woman** in cardiac arrest, high-quality CPR with manual uterine displacement, early ALS and emergent delivery of the foetus if early return of spontaneous circulation (ROSC) is not achieved remain key interventions.

Foetal survival usually depends on maternal survival and initial resuscitation efforts should focus on the pregnant mother.

From 20 weeks' gestation, the uterus can compress the inferior vena cava (IVC) and aorta, impeding venous return and cardiac output and therefore can cause pre-arrest hypotension or shock and, in the critically ill patient, may precipitate cardiac arrest [47, [49]]. During cardiac arrest, the compromise in venous return and cardiac output by the gravid uterus limits the effectiveness of chest compressions. Manually displace the uterus to the left is recommended to reduce IVC compression.

During CPR, the hand position for chest compressions may need to be slightly higher on the sternum for patients with advanced pregnancy—third trimester [48].

During BLS and ALS, pregnant patients are at risk of aspiration and oxygenation and ventilation are the priority over aspiration prevention. Early tracheal intubation (using a tracheal tube 0.5–1 mm internal diameter smaller than that used for a non-pregnant woman) with mechanical ventilation will however make ventilation of the lungs easier in the presence of increased intra-abdominal pressure.

The 4Hs and 4Ts approach helps identify all the common causes of cardiac arrest in pregnancy. The most important causes are

- Haemorrhage: postpartum haemorrhage, ectopic pregnancy, placental abruption, placenta praevia, placenta accrete, uterine rupture. The key steps for treatment are stop the bleeding, fluid resuscitation, including use of rapid transfusion system and cell salvage [50] and correction of coagulopathy including use of tranexamic acid and/or recombinant activated factor VII.
- Cardiovascular disease: acute myocardial infarction and aneurysm or dissection of the aorta and peripartum cardiomyopathy, pulmonary embolism, amniotic fluid embolism cause most deaths from acquired cardiac disease.
- Pre-eclampsia and eclampsia need magnesium sulphate infusion for the treatment in peri-arrest situation.

Consider the need for an emergency hysterectomy or Caesarean section as soon as a pregnant woman goes into cardiac arrest. Delivery will relieve IVC compression and may improve chances of maternal resuscitation. Seek for help and ask gynaecologist and neonatologist to start preparing for emergency caesarean section—the foetus will need to be delivered if initial resuscitation efforts fail. The caesarean delivery also enables access to the infant so that newborn resuscitation can begin [4].

Elderly people have an increased incidence of cardiac causes of arrest because the incidence of coronary heart disease and chronic heart failure increases with age. The incidence of PEA as the first recorded rhythm increases significantly with age with a decrease of the incidence of shockable rhythms (VF/pulseless VT) [4]. No modifications of standard resuscitation protocols are needed for aged patients in cardiac arrest. Rescuers should be aware that the risk of both sternal and rib fractures is higher in elderly and the incidence of CPR-related injuries increases with duration of CPR [51]. When deciding to resuscitate elderly patients, age alone should not be the element to consider and other more established criteria (witnessed arrest, resuscitation times, first recorded rhythm, the degree of autonomy, quality of life, mental status and presence of major comorbidities) are important factors. Whenever possible, a decision to resuscitate or not should be discussed in advance with the patient and his family.

Special circumstances in cardiac arrest need special interventions with an appropriate approach of guidelines for cardiopulmonary resuscitation.

Author details

Diana Carmen Cimpoesu[1,2*] and Tudor Ovidiu Popa[1,2]

*Address all correspondence to: dcimpoiesu@yahoo.com

1 University of Medicine and Pharmacy Gr.T.Popa, Iasi, Romania

2 Emergency Department, Emergency County Hospital Sf.Spiridon, Iasi, Romania

References

[1] Cimpoesu D. [coordinator], Rotaru L, Petris A et al. Current protocols and guidelines in emergency medicine. UMF "Gr. T. Popa" Publishing House, Iasi 2011.

[2] Nikolaos Nikolaou, Maaret Castrén, Koenraad G. Monsieurs, Diana Cimpoesu, Marios Georgiou, Violetta Raffay, Rudolph Koster, Silvija Hunyadi-Anticevi, Anatolij Truhlárˇ, Leo Bossaert, The EUROCALL investigators. Time delays to reach dispatch centres in different regions in Europe. Are we losing the window of opportunity? — The EUROCALL study. Resuscitation 111 [2017] 8-13

[3] Jan-Thorsten Gräsner, Leo L.Bossaert, Diana Cimpoesu et al., EuReCa ONE – 27 Nations, ONE Europe, ONE Registry. A prospective one month analysis of out-of-hospital cardiac arrest outcomes in 27 countries in Europe, Resuscitation, Vol. 105:188-195, http://dx.doi.org/10.1016/j.resuscitation.2016.06.004

[4] European R7esuscitation Council Guidelines for Resuscitation 2015, Truhlář A, Barelli, Al et al. Resuscitation, Volume 95, 148-201

[5] Soar J, Perkins GD, Abbas G, et al. European Resuscitation Council Guidelines for Resuscitation 2010 Section 8. Cardiac arrest in special circumstances: electrolyte abnormalities, poisoning, drowning, accidental hypothermia, hyperthermia, asthma, anaphylaxis, cardiac surgery, trauma, pregnancy, electrocution. Resuscitation 2010;**81**:1400-33.

[6] Judith E. Tintinalli, et. al.-Tintinalli's Emergency Medicine A Comprehensive Study Guide, 8th edition McGraw-Hill Publishing House, NewYork, 2016, ISBN: 007179476X

[7] Lexow K. Severe accidental hypothermia: survival after 6 hours 30 minutes of cardiopulmonary resuscitation. Arctic Med Res 1991;**50**:112-4.44.

[8] Pasquier M, Zurron N, Weith B, et al. Deep accidental hypothermia with coretemperature below 24 degrees c presenting with vital signs. High Alt Med Biol 2014;**15**:58-63.

[9] Wood S. Interactions between hypoxia and hypothermia. Annu Rev Physiol 1991;**53**:71-85.

[10] Simpson CR, Sheikh A. Adrenaline is first line treatment for the emergency treatment of anaphylaxis. Resuscitation 2010;**81**:641-2.

[11] Kleber C, Giesecke MT, Lindner T, Haas NP, Buschmann CT. Requirement for a structured algorithm in cardiac arrest following major trauma: epidemiology, management errors, and preventability of traumatic deaths in Berlin. Resuscitation 2014;**85**:405-10.

[12] Warner KJ, Copass MK, Bulger EM. Paramedic use of needle thoracostomy inthe prehospital environment. Prehosp Emerg Care 2008;**12**:162-8.

[13] Escott ME, Gleisberg GR, Kimmel K, Karrer A, Cosper J, Monroe BJ. Simple thoracostomy. Moving beyond needle decompression in traumatic cardiac arrest. JEMS 2014;**39**:26-32.

[14] Pokorna M, Necas E, Skripsky R, Kratochvil J, Andrlik M, Franek O. How accurately can the aetiology of cardiac arrest be established in an out-of-hospital setting? Analysis by "concordance in diagnosis crosscheck tables". Resuscitation 2011;**82**:391-7

[15] Cimpoesu D Pulmonary Thromboembolism : prehospital and Emergencu Department approach in Petris A, Tînt D, Tatu-Chitoiu G, Pop C [coordinator]. Pulmonary thromboembolism: a modern approche. Ed. PIM, Iasi 2015

[16] Cimpoesu D, Petris A, Tatu-Chitoiu G, Pop C, Tînt D. ESC 2008 Guidelines for diagnosis and treatment of pulmonary embolism – vademecum for Emergency Department. Edited by Sandesc D, Bedreag O, Papurica M. in Recommendations and protocols in anesthesia, intensive care and emergency medicine 2010, Mirton Publishing House, Timisoara 2010:533-550. ISBN 978-973-52-0914-8

[17] Cimpoesu D, Rotaru L, Diaconu C, Petris O, Petris A. Protocol approach to chest pain in emergency. Edited by Sandesc D, Bedreag O, Papurica M in Recommendations and protocols in anesthesia, intensive care and emergency medicine, Mirton Publishing House, Timisoara 2009:591-614. ISBN 978-973-52-0736-6

[18] Tatu-Chitoiu G, Dorobantu M, Petris A, Deleanu D, Arafat R, Cizmaru O, Cimpoesu D, Georgescu V, Oprisan M, Dimitriu I, PopescuL, Costinas M, Oprita B. Guidelines for diagnosis and treatment in pre-hospital phase of acute myocardial infarction with ST segment elevation. Curtea Veche Publishing House, Bucharest 2009. ISBN 978-973-1983-14-1, 216p

[19] Petris AO, Tatu-Chitoiu G, Cimpoesu D, Costache I, Tînt D.Thrombolysis for intra-hospital cardiac arrest related to pulmonary embolism-study design. Biomedical Research 2017;**28**(1):106-110

[20] Bottiger BW, Arntz HR, Chamberlain DA, et al. Thrombolysis during resuscitation for out-of-hospital cardiac arrest. N Engl J Med 2008;**359**:2651-62

[21] Mowry JB, Spyker DA, Cantilena Jr LR, McMillan N, Ford M. 2013 Annual Report of the American Association of Poison Control Centers' National Poison Data System [NPDS]: 31st Annual Report. Clin Toxicol [Phila] 2014;**52**:1032-283.

[22] Nunnally ME, O'Connor MF, Kordylewski H, Westlake B, Dutton RP. The incidence and risk factors for perioperative cardiac arrest observed in the national anesthesia clinical outcomes registry. Anesth Analg 2015;**120**:364-70

[23] Sprung J, Warner ME, Contreras MG, et al. Predictors of survival following cardiac arrest in patients undergoing noncardiac surgery: a study of 518,294 patients at a tertiary referral center. Anesthesiology 2003;**99**:259-69.

[24] Newland MC, Ellis SJ, Lydiatt CA, et al. Anesthetic-related cardiac arrest and its mortality: a report covering 72,959 anesthetics over 10 years from a US teaching hospital. Anesthesiology 2002;**97**:108-15.

[25] Davis TR, Young BA, Eisenberg MS, Rea TD, Copass MK, Cobb LA. Outcome of cardiac arrests attended by emergency medical services staff at community outpatient dialysis centers. Kidney international 2008;**73**:933-9.

[26] Lafrance JP, Nolin L, Senecal L, Leblanc M. Predictors and outcome of cardiopulmonary resuscitation [CPR] calls in a large haemodialysis unit over a seven-year period. Nephrol Dial Transplant 2006;**21**:1006-12.

[27] Meaney PA, Nadkarni VM, Kern KB, Indik JH, Halperin HR, Berg RA. Rhythms and outcomes of adult in-hospital cardiac arrest. Critical care medicine 2010;**38**:101-8.

[28] Girotra S, Nallamothu BK, Spertus JA, et al. Trends in survival after in-hospital cardiac arrest. The New England journal of medicine 2012;**367**:1912-20.

[29] Bird S, Petley GW, Deakin CD, Clewlow F. Defibrillation during renal dialysis: a survey of UK practice and procedural recommendations. Resuscitation 2007;**73**:347-53.

[30] Perkins GD, Stephenson BT, Smith CM, Gao F. A comparison between over-the-head and standard cardiopulmonary resuscitation. Resuscitation 2004;**61**:155-61.

[31] Handley AJ, Handley JA. Performing chest compressions in a confined space. Resuscitation 2004;**61**:55-61.

[32] Maisch S, Issleib M, Kuhls B, et al. A comparison between over-the-head and standard cardiopulmonary resuscitation performed by two rescuers: a simulation study. The Journal of emergency medicine. 2010;**39**:369-76.

[33] Hung KK, Cocks RA, Poon WK, Chan EY, Rainer TH, Graham CA. Medical volunteers in commercial flight medical diversions. Aviat Space Environ Med. 2013;**84**:491-7.

[34] Lyon RM, Nelson MJ. Helicopter emergency medical services [HEMS] response to out-of-hospital cardiac arrest. Scandinavian journal of trauma, resuscitation and emergency medicine 2013;**21**:1.

[35] Brugger H, Paal P, Boyd J. Prehospital resuscitation of the buried avalanche victim. High Alt Med Biol 2011;**12**:199-205.

[36] Wang JC, Tsai SH, Chen YL, et al. The physiological effects and quality of chest compressions during CPR at sea level and high altitude. Am J Emerg Med 2014;**32**:1183-8.

[37] Tomazin I, Ellerton J, Reisten O, Soteras I, Avbelj M, International Commission for Mountain Emergency Medicine. Medical standards for mountain rescue operations using helicopters: official consensus recommendations of the International Commission for Mountain Emergency Medicine [ICAR MEDCOM].High Alt Med Biol 2011;**12**:335-41.

[38] Fahmy FS, Brinsden MD, Smith J, Frame JD. Lightning: the multisystem group injuries. The Journal of trauma 1999;**46**:937-40.

[39] Browne BJ, Gaasch WR. Electrical injuries and lightning. Emerg Med Clin North Am 1992;**10**:211-29.

[40] Kleiner JP, Wilkin JH. Cardiac effects of lightning stroke. Jama 1978;**240**:2757-9.

[41] Lichtenberg R, Dries D, Ward K, Marshall W, Scanlon P. Cardiovascular effects of lightning strikes. J Am Coll Cardiol 1993;**21**:531-6.

[42] SALT mass casualty triage: concept endorsed by the American College of Emergency Physicians, American College of Surgeons Committee on Trauma, American Trauma Society, National Association of EMS Physicians, National Disaster Life Support Education Consortium, and State and Territorial Injury Prevention Directors Association. Disaster Med Public Health Prep 2008;**2**:245-6.

[43] Lim WJ, Mohammed Akram R, Carson KV, et al. Non-invasive positive pressure ventilation for treatment of respiratory failure due to severe acute exacerbations of asthma. The Cochrane database of systematic reviews 2012;**12**:CD004360.

[44] Leatherman JW, McArthur C, Shapiro RS. Effect of prolongation of expiratory time on dynamic hyperinflation in mechanically ventilated patients with severe asthma. Critical care medicine 2004;**32**:1542-5.

[45] Deakin CD, McLaren RM, Petley GW, Clewlow F, Dalrymple-Hay MJ. Effects of positive end-expiratory pressure on transthoracic impedance-- implications for defibrillation. Resuscitation 1998;**37**:9-12.

[46] Hubner P, Meron G, Kurkciyan I, et al. Neurologic causes of cardiac arrest and outcomes. The Journal of emergency medicine 2014;**47**:660-7.

[47] Page-Rodriguez A, Gonzalez-Sanchez JA. Perimortem cesarean section of twin pregnancy: case report and review of the literature. Academic emergency medicine : official journal of the Society for Academic Emergency Medicine 1999;**6**:1072-4.

[48] Lipman S, Cohen S, Einav S, et al. The Society for Obstetric Anesthesia and Perinatology consensus statement on the management of cardiac arrest in pregnancy. Anesthesia and analgesia 2014;**118**:1003-16.

[49] Nolan JP, Soar J, Wenzel V, Paal P. Cardiopulmonary resuscitation and management of cardiac arrest. Nat Rev Cardiol 2012;**9**:499-511.

[50] Geoghegan J, Daniels JP, Moore PA, Thompson PJ, Khan KS, Gulmezoglu AM. Cell salvage at caesarean section: the need for an evidence-based approach. BJOG 2009;**116**:743-7.

[51] Kashiwagi Y, Sasakawa T, Tampo A, et al. Computed tomography findings of complications resulting from cardiopulmonary resuscitation. Resuscitation 2015;**88**:86-91.

Chapter 3

Resuscitation of Obstetric Patient

Daniel Molano Franco and María Velez Maya

Additional information is available at the end of the chapter

http://dx.doi.org/10.5772/intechopen.68420

Abstract

The number of cases of pregnant patients with cardiorespiratory arrest requiring resuscitation has increased worldwide, secondary to the main number of patients with high-risk pregnancies associated with chronic, especially cardiopulmonary, pathologies. The knowledge of the resuscitation algorithms by the health personnel responsible for the care of pregnant patients is mandatory, because due to different physiological and anatomical changes, there are particularities in the management and use of medications. In addition, a detailed description of the steps included in the resuscitation is necessary, where assessment of the airway, ventilation, circulation, and defibrillation determines a step in resuscitation. One of the determining and exclusive events in this type of patients is cesarea perimortem. That is why it includes a concrete description of the time and the indications for its realization. Finally, a list of medicines most used in resuscitation in pregnancy, with its dosage and safety range, is mentioned. The pregnant patient poses a challenge to resuscitation teams. This review refers to the recommendations for establishing "obstetric blue code" protocols at the institutional level.

Keywords: reanimation, maternal arrest, pregnancy, cardiopulmonary, perimortem caesarean

1. Introduction

The approach to resuscitation in pregnancy determines several conditions that go from the physiological, anatomical, and emotional point of view, as we face a catastrophic event and the challenge of restoring the health condition of two living beings as a mother [1]. Knowledge and training in resuscitation of the obstetric patient has had a great development in the last decade, with an increasing number of publications and special chapters in the international guides of resuscitation [2].

Although maternal mortality worldwide has declined by 44%, there has been a worrying increase in extreme maternal morbidity and mortality in developed countries around the world due to increased pregnancy age and comorbidities that determine a greater number of situations of cardiac arrest [3].

In the USA, the prevalence of events requiring cardiac resuscitation in hospitalized obstetric patients was 8.5 × 100,000, with a survival rate of only 59% in the mother [4].

We believe that the scope of this chapter includes the knowledge of the various groups responsible for mother–child resuscitation, such as emergency physicians, obstetricians, anesthesiologists, critical care physicians, and neonatologists, as well as nurses and midwives.

2. Changes physiologic in the mother

The physiological and anatomical changes of pregnancy require some modifications in the resuscitation protocols, these changes begin early in pregnancy, reach their peak during the second trimester, and then, remain relatively constant until delivery.

The major hemodynamic changes induced by pregnancy include an increase in cardiac output between 30 and 40% (as a result of increased stroke volume and to a lesser extent increased maternal heart rate 15–20 bpm) [5], plasma volume expansion is 10–15% at 6–12 weeks of gestation, and at the term, is 30–50% higher than non-pregnant women, increase in red cell volume [6] (a greater increase in intravascular volume than red cell mass, that results in the dilutional or physiologic anemia of pregnancy), reductions in systemic vascular resistance and systemic blood pressure [7].

Most of the increase in cardiac output is distributed in the placenta, kidneys, and skin so that the mechanical effects of the gravid uterus can decrease venous return from the inferior vena cava and obstruct blood flow through the abdominal aorta; all of above, contribute to unsuccessful cardiopulmonary resuscitation. Left lateral uterine displacement is necessary in the pregnant patient with fundal height at or above the umbilicus, to minimize aortocaval compression, to optimize venous return, and to generate adequate stroke volume during cardiopulmonary resuscitation [6].

During pregnancy, the anatomy of the upper respiratory airway undergoes numerous changes; upper airway, the pharynx and larynx edema occur as a result of hormonal effects and may reduce visualization during laryngoscopy and therefore, intubation in a pregnant woman can be difficult, and smaller endotracheal tubes may be needed [6, 8]. Therefore, progesterone relaxes gastroesophageal sphincters and prolongs transit times throughout the intestinal tract, predisposing the patient to aspiration of stomach contents [9].

Changes in the thorax and abdomen appear early in pregnancy; even before displacement from the enlarging uterus. In the first trimester, the subcostal angle changes from 68 to 103°, the diaphragm rises by up to 4 cm and the chest diameter increases by 2 cm or more, diaphragmatic excursion increases by up to 2 cm (the result is "barrel chested" appearance) [8].

Since the first trimester of pregnancy, a relative hyperventilation occurs, with minute ventilation rise by 50% at term, mediated by the elevated serum progesterone levels. This produces a mild respiratory alkalosis with compensatory renal excretion of bicarbonate [8].

The functional residual capacity decreases approximately 20% due to the upward shift in the diaphragm as the uterus enlarges, while oxygen consumption increases by 20% during pregnancy to meet the increased oxygen demands of the placenta, fetus and maternal organs. These two factors are responsible for hypoventilation in the pregnant woman [5, 9].

Forced expiratory volume (FEV1) does not change during pregnancy, but expiratory reserve volume and residual volume decrease, inspiratory capacity is mildly increased, resulting in a minimal drop in the total lung capacity from 4.2 to 4 l, In addition, there is a decrease in arterial carbon dioxide ($PaCO_2$) levels from 40 mmHg in non-pregnant to 27–32 mmHg during pregnancy, so that, the resultant arterial pH is normal to slightly alkalotic (between 7.40 and 7.45). The decrease in $PaCO_2$ helps the fetus to eliminate carbon dioxide across the placenta [9].

3. Etiology

It is necessary to know the possible etiology of cardiac arrest in pregnant women to identify and treat correctly the causal factors and therefore give the mother and the fetus a better chance of survival. The cause of maternal cardiac arrest can often be multifactorial, and in many cases it is associated with chronic health problems that exist before pregnancy, so women with comorbidities should have multidisciplinary follow-up. Even so, it must be taken into account that cardiorespiratory arrest (CRA) in pregnant women occurs frequently in previously healthy woman in relation to hemorrhage or embolism (non-arrhythmogenic causes, unlike non-pregnant women). This refers to the non-pulsed electrical activity algorithm (AESP) in which the modified 5H and 5T must be remembered (see **Table 1**) [4, 10–15].

5H	5T
1. *Hypoxia*: particular predisposition that the pregnant woman has due to the high consumption of oxygen by the developing fetus	1. Toxics/tablets
2. *Hypovolemia*: uterine atony, placental abruption, placenta previa, placenta accreta, subcapsular hepatic hematoma, ectopic pregnancy, uterine rupture, retained products of conception	2. *Thrombosis*: pulmonary thrombosis and Coronary thrombosis
3. *Hydroelectrolitic*: hypermagnesemia. Treatment of threatened preterm or preeclampsia, particularly in renal failure, hyperkalemia/hypokalemia	3. *Tension*: pneumothorax tension
4. Hydrogenions-acidosis	4. *Tamponade*: cardiac tamponade.
5. Hypothermia	5. Trauma

Table 1. Etiologies of maternal arrest (5H-5T) [11–15].

The main causes of CRA in pregnant women include bleeding, heart failure, sepsis, and amniotic fluid embolism, and the main causes of mortality in this population are the cardiac disease, sepsis, preeclampsia/eclampsia, hemorrhage, cerebrovascular events, amniotic fluid embolism, complications from anesthesia, and thrombosis/thromboembolism [4, 10]. A way to remember those causes is the mnemonic of the American Heart Association (AHA), because the obstetrics' CRA causes are different from the general population [5] (see **Table 2**).

Letter	Meaning	Etiology
A	Anesthetic Accidents	High neuraxial block Hypotension Loss of airway Aspiration Respiratory depression Local anesthetic systemic toxicity Trauma Suicide
B	Bleeding	Coagulopathy Uterine atony Placenta accreta Placental abruption Placenta previa Retained products of conception Uterine rupture Surgical Transfusion reaction
C	Cardiovascular	Myocardial infarction Aortic dissection Cardiomyopathy Arrhythmias Valve disease Congenital heart disease
D	Drugs	Oxytocin-magnesium-opioids-insulin Drug error Illicit drugs Anaphylaxis
E	Embolic	Amniotic fluid embolus Pulmonary embolus Cerebrovascular event Venous air embolism
F	Fever	Infection/sepsis
G	General	H's and T's (**Table 1**)
H	Hypertension	Preeclampsia-eclampsia HELLP syndrome Intracranial bleed

Table 2. Etiologies of maternal arrest (A to H's mnemonic) [5].

http://dx.doi.org/10.5772/intechopen.68420

4. Management

The management of CRA in pregnant women should ideally be performed by trained individuals, with knowledge of the physiological changes in pregnancy, in the centers where the equipments necessary for cesarean perimortem and for neonatal resuscitation are available. The most important pillar in the management of CRA in pregnant women is prevention [5], guaranteeing adequate oxygenation, and circulatory volume, so it is recommended to place the patient in a position of complete left lateral decubitus to relieve the aortocava compression, administration of 100% oxygen by face mask to treat or prevent hypoxemia, establish intravenous access above the diaphragm to ensure intravenous therapy is not obstructed by the pregnant uterus and to investigate and treat precipitating factors [11]. In the CRA there is basic and advanced management, first the basic management of pregnant women in CRA and then the advanced management will be discussed, emphasizing the changes with respect to the CRA of the non-pregnant adult.

4.1. Basic cardiovascular life support

the basic life support (BLS), the first responders must initiate usual resuscitation measures, including board placement, and provision of chest compressions and appropriate airway management, defibrillation where appropriate, and manual left uterine displacement [12] (algorithm N1). A minimum of four responders must be present to carry out all tasks effectively (**Figure 1**).

4.1.1. Circulation

Thoracic compressions: the patient should be placed supine for chest compressions (chest compressions performed with the patient in a tilt could be significantly less effective than those performed with the patient in the usual supine position, and this could have a major impact on the chance of successful resuscitation), which must be effective at least 5 cm deep, are performed 3 cm above the traditional sternal point, frequently at least 100 per min and with a sequentiality of 30 chest compressions: 2 artificial ventilation, deviation of the uterus to the left manually, it is recommended to allow complete thoracic expansion after each compression and to minimize interruptions in chest compressions. Once a device has been placed the compressions can be continuous and not alternate with the ventilation [10–12]. There is no literature examining the use of mechanical chest compressions in pregnancy, and this is not advised at this time. Previous guidelines recommended placing the hands slightly higher on the sternum in the pregnant patient, but there are no scientific data to support this recommendation.

4.1.2. Airway

After placing the pregnant woman in a suitable position, the opening of the airway is performed, head extension maneuver is performed, neck flexion and chin elevation (except in patients with a history of cervical trauma, in which if only the lower jaw is raised), if there is

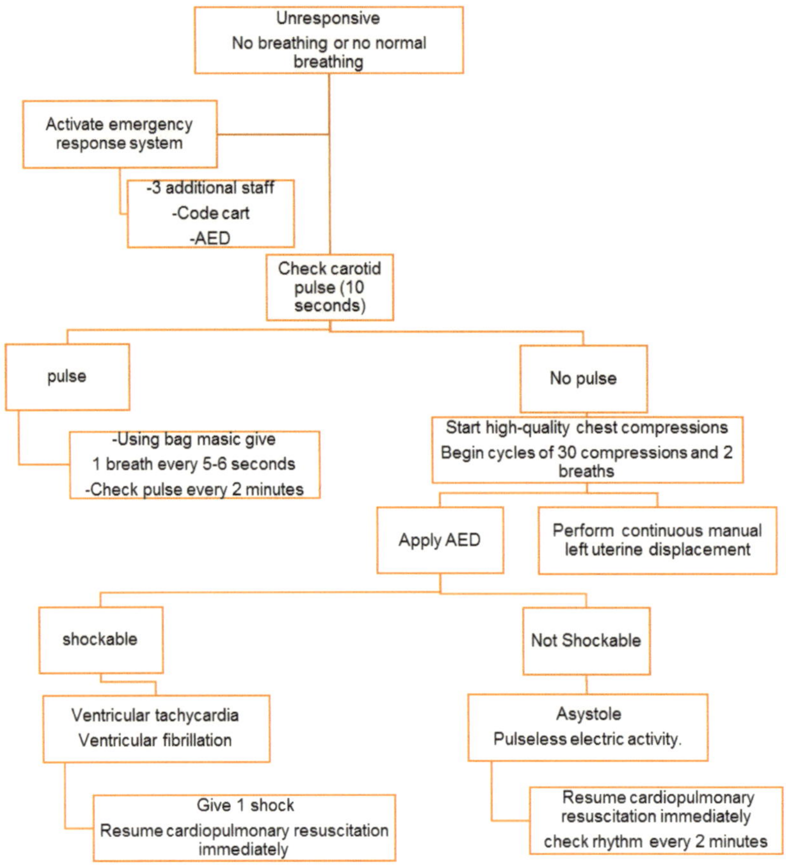

Figure 1. Basic life support (BLS)—cardiac arrest in pregnancy.

no response, be prepared to ensure the airway definitively, initiate with pre-oxygenation of the patient with 100% FiO_2, due to the complications in the pregnant patient because of the physiological changes of the pregnancy. It is recommended to perform this procedure with personnel having greater training in airways, it is recommended to have the "STUBBY" (short-handled) laryngoscope for mammary hypertrophy, and to have on hand a difficult airway equipment with elements such as mask Laryngeal in case conventional intubation is not possible. It is recommended to make only one attempt and ask for help from the most qualified personnel, if you are in second or third level of care, request help from the anesthesiology group.

4.1.3. Defibrillation

Identify the defibrillator of your workplace and identify if it is biphasic or monophasic. In the absence of a biphasic defibrillator, it is acceptable to use a single-phase, so far has not shown any injury to the fetus by defibrillation. Defibrillary Cardiopulmonary Arrest (CPA) Rates: We recommend the administration of 200 J by a biphasic defibrillator or 360 J by a single-phase defibrillator in ventricular fibrillation and non-pulse ventricular tachycardia, alternating with the administration of the following drugs: Adrenaline 1 mg IV every 3 min [10–14]. The energy required for defibrillation during cardiac arrest in pregnancy would be the same as the most current recommendations for the non-pregnant patient.

5. Advanced cardiovascular life support

Although current guidelines for management of CPA adults say that chest compressions should not be interrupted initially for ventilation or airway placement. The pregnant patient has a very limited oxygen reserve and requires early attention to airways and ventilation.

In the advanced cardiovascular life support (ACLS), it is recommended that endotracheal intubation should be performed by an experienced laryngoscopist (not more than two laryngoscopy attempts should be made and prolonged intubation attempts should be avoided to prevent deoxygenation, prolonged interruption in chest compressions, airway trauma, and bleeding), and starting with an endotracheal tube with a 6.0–7.0 mm inner diameter is recommended, because the glottis in pregnancy is often smaller for edema. The cricoid pressure is not routinely recommended, but, continuous waveform capnography, in addition to clinical assessment, is recommended as the most reliable method of confirming and monitoring correct placement of the endotracheal tube (**Figure 2**).

If attempts at airway control fail and mask ventilation is not possible, current guidelines for emergency invasive airway should be followed.

Given the lethality of cardiopulmonary arrest, the benefits from use outweigh any possible fetal risks. All medications at the same doses for treatment of cardiopulmonary arrest in the non-pregnant patient are used for the pregnant patient (**Table 3**).

5.1. Arrhythmia-specific therapy during cardiac arrest

5.1.1. Cardiopulmonary non-defibrillation rhythms

In case of asystole and pulseless electrical activity, focus on chest compressions as well as drug administration. Other potentially lethal arrhythmias that should be treated.

5.1.2. Ventricular tachycardia with pulse

Stable monomorphic VT with adult pulse responds well to biphasic or monophasic (synchronized) cardioversion discharges at initial doses of 100 J. If there is no adequate response after the first discharge, it is reasonable to increase the dose in a staggered manner.

5.1.3. Supraventricular paroxysmal tachycardia

In addition to synchronous cardioversion, adenosine is also recommended as a safe and potentially effective drug. There are no data yet on pregnancy. The recommended initial

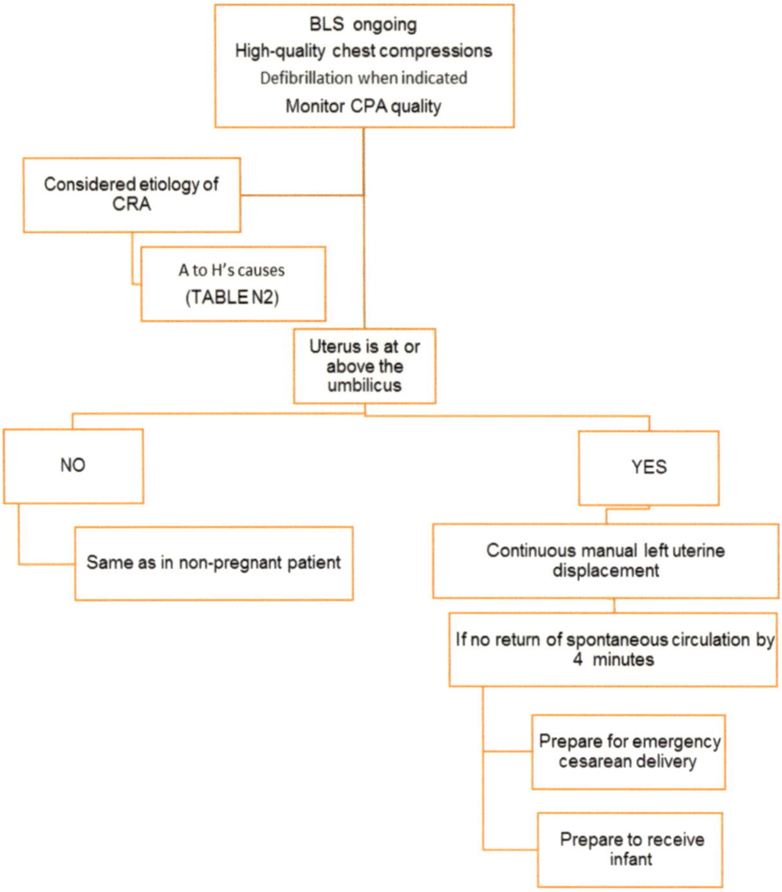

Figure 2. Advanced cardiovascular life support (ACLS)—cardiac arrest in pregnancy.

Medications	Use	Adverse effects	Observations	Dose
Epinephrine	If VF or VT persists after at least one attempt at defibrillation and 2 min of CPA	Reduce uterine blood flow through alpha-adrenergic-mediated blood vessel vasoconstriction	Is superior	1 mg IV every 3–5 min
Vasopressin	Was removed from the treatment algorithm for CPA	Uterine contractions	Is not clearly superior to epinephrine	Is not recommended
Magnesium sulfate Pregnancy	• Prevention of eclamptic seizures • Fetal neuroprotection before preterm delivery	Magnesium toxicity	Should be discontinued Calcium chloride (10 mL of a 10% solution) or calcium gluconate (30 mL of a 10% solution) intravenously or intraosseously	4 or 6 g IV, followed by a maintenance 1–2 g IV/h

Medications	Use	Adverse effects	Observations	Dose
CPA	• Polymorphic VT consistent with torsade de pointes		Is not recommended for routine use in adult cardiac arrest patients	2 g IV, followed by a maintenance infusion
Sodium bicarbonate	Correction of maternal acidosis	May worsen fetal acidosis Since crosses the placenta, overcorrection of maternal acidosis will lead to pooling of carbon dioxide in the fetal compartment	Guidelines do not recommend routine use Useful in life-threatening hyperkalemia or tricyclic antidepressant overdose	1–2 mEq/kg IV
Amiodarone	Primary drug in the arrhythmia treatment algorithm VF or VT unresponsive to defibrillation, CPA, and epinephrine	• Hypothyroidism or hyperthyroidism in the mother or fetus because of the iodine in amiodarone • Fetal bradycardia • Fetal QT interval prolongation • Premature labor • Low birth weight	Neonates of mothers taking amiodarone should have complete thyroid function tests and developmental follow-up	300 mg IV with a repeat dose of 150 mg IV as indicated

Table 3. Medications used in CPA and its consequences in pregnancy.

biphasic energy dose for synchronous cardioversion of atrial fibrillation is 120–200 J. The initial monophasic dose for synchronous cardioversion of atrial fibrillation is 200 J. In general, atrial flutter cardioversion and other supraventricular rhythms require less energy. An initial energy of 50–100 J with a single-phase or biphasic device is usually sufficient. If the first discharge of the cardioversion fails, the dose should be increased stepwise.

6. Modifications of the basic support and advanced cardiac life support in pregnancy

The three major modifications during the pregnant patient CPR are given in below sections.

6.1. Shift of the uterus to the left at 15–30° and upward during chest compressions

To improve placental perfusion and enable a perimortem cesarean, it has been described that thoracic compressions in non-pregnant patients produce 30% of the CG, to which 25% more is added by applying the lateralization of the uterus to the left. For this purpose, a blanket can be placed under the right hip or the Cardiff resuscitation wedge, which maintains the patient in the left dorsal decubitus position at 27° since an inclination greater than 30° has been associated with a significant decrease in force generation during chest compression.

6.2. Early endotracheal intubation

Waive ventilation with bag-mask and proceed directly to endotracheal intubation by the most experienced person, as the physiological changes of pregnancy increase 10 times the risk of complications they put. It is life-threatening mainly because of decreased functional residual capacity (CRF) by compression of the pregnant uterus, resulting in rapid desaturation, as well as edema (often thin tubes are used) and hyperaemia of the upper airway which cause frequent bleeding and make it difficult to visualize the vocal cords, especially in the presence of preeclampsia. In addition, decreased gastric motility and relaxation of esophageal sphincter tone increase the risk of aspiration. For all of the above, it is also recommended the use of muscle relaxants and rapid intubation sequence (SIR), as well as nasogastric tube placement (SNG) [12–14].

6.3. Cesarean perimortem

Cesarean perimortem is defined as the birth of the fetus after maternal cardiac arrest. Birth is almost always accomplished through cesarean delivery, but assisted vaginal delivery is appropriate if the cervix is fully dilated and the neonate is at a low station and can be delivered within 5 min of maternal cardiorespiratory collapse [15]. A review of published cases up to 2010 has showed that the cesarean perimortem led to a clear maternal survival benefit 31.7% [16].

The purpose of the cesarean perimortem is twofold. The first is facilitation of resuscitation, relieving aortocaval compression by emptying the uterus significantly improves resuscitative efforts. Second, early delivery of the baby, is accomplished with a decreased risk of permanent neurological damage from anoxia.

It is contemplated within the "four-five rule" of obstetric stop, which consists of starting the cesarean section 4 min after the maternal cardiac arrest so that he drinks be born within 5 min after the arrest spontaneous circulation and not later, especially when the cause is irreversible (e.g. abrupt), which in turn improves the maternal GC by 30% with autotransfusion of 500 ml. It is the most important consideration in the OP. According to Katz, 71% of babies surviving maternal cardiorespiratory arrest with good neurologic outcome were removed in 5 min or less. Therefore, fetal extraction is considered as the "D" of cardiopulmonary resuscitation in the pregnant woman.

Sudden substantial improvement in hemodynamics with a return of pulse and blood pressure immediately after perimortem cesarean delivery has been observed.

There are three pathophysiological states (in relation to the uterus and navel): O Pregnancy < 20 weeks, AU below navel: impaired hemodynamic compromise for the mother by the uterus, non-viable baby. No benefit of cesarean perimortem.

Or pregnancy of 20–23 weeks, AU up to 3 cm above the navel: possible hemodynamic involvement of the mother by the uterus, probably not viable baby. Consider cesarean perimortem to save the life of the mother.

O pregnancy ≥ 24 weeks, AU at 4 cm above the navel: possible hemodynamic compromise exerted by the uterus, cesarean section perimortem is indicated during cardiopulmonary arrest to benefit the mother as well as the fetus. Consider not closing the abdominal incision if cesarean section was necessary, to bind blood vessels as well as reduce the possibility of an abdominal compartment syndrome [2, 3, 6–10].

If the cesarean perimortem could not be performed by the 5-min mark, it was still advisable to prepare to evacuate the uterus while the resuscitation continued, infant survival has been seen even when delivery occurred > 5 min from the onset of maternal cardiac arrest. Neonatal survival was documented even when delivery occurred up to 30 min after the onset of maternal cardiac arrest [17]. The procedure should be performed at the site of the maternal resuscitation. Time should not be wasted in moving the patient or waiting for surgical equipment or doing abdominal preparation [18]. The only equipment needed to start is a scalpel [5].

7. Other considerations

- Regarding the drugs used in a cardiorespiratory arrest, these do not differ in the pregnant patient, although it is recognized that the vasopressors could decrease the uterine blood flow, remember that the best possibility for the survival of the fetus is the survival of the mother.
- Regarding the energy used for defibrillation/cardioversion, pregnancy does not significantly alter the electrical impedance of the chest wall and no deleterious effect of maternal defibrillation/cardioversion has been reported in newborns.
- Oxytocin and prostaglandins may be considered to correct uterine atony.
- In summary, an Obstetric Code (OC) is a situation in which a doctor can save two lives as long as resources are available and procedures are performed in less than 5 min [15, 19, 20].

Author details

Daniel Molano Franco[1]* and María Velez Maya[2]

*Address all correspondence to: dalemofra@gmail.com

1 Gynecology and Obstetric, Intensive Care Medicine University Clinic Colombia, Bogotá, Colombia

2 Gynecology and Obstetrics, University National of Colombia, Bogotá, Colombia

References

[1] Cantwell R, Clutton-Brock T, Cooper G, et al. "Saving mothers' lives: Reviewing maternal deaths to make motherhood safer: 2006-2008. The eighth report of the confidential enquiries into maternal deaths in the United Kingdom." British Journal of Obstetrics and Gynaecology. 2011;**118**(1):1-203

[2] Neumar RW, Otto CW, Link MS, et al. Part 8: Adult advanced cardiovascular life support: 2010 American Heart Association guidelines for cardiopulmonary resuscitation and emergency cardiovascular care. Circulation. 2010;**122**(Suppl 3):S729–S767

[3] Trends in maternal mortality: 1990 to 2013. Estimates by WHO, UNICEF, UNFPA, the World Bank and the United Nations Population Division. Geneva (Switzerland): World Health Organization; 2014

[4] Mhyre JM, Tsen LC, Einav S, et al. Cardiac arrest during hospitalization for delivery in the United States, 1998-2011. Anesthesiology. 2014;**120**:810-818

[5] Jeejeebhoy FM, Zelop CM, Lipman S, et al. Cardiac arrest in pregnancy: A scientific statement from the American Heart Association. Circulation. 2015;**132**:1747-1773

[6] Tan EK, Tan EL. Alterations in physiology and anatomy during pregnancy. Best practice & research. Clinical Obstetrics & Gynaecology. 2013;**27**:791-802. DOI: 10.1016/j. bpobgyn. 2013.08.001

[7] Melchiorre K, Sharma R, Thilaganathan B. Cardiac structure and function in normal pregnancy. Current Opinion in Obstetrics & Gynecology. 2012;**24**(6):413-421

[8] Hegewald MJ, Crapo RO. Respiratory physiology in pregnancy. Clinics in Chest Medicine. 2011;**32**(1):1-13

[9] Carlin A, Alfirevic Z. Physiological changes of pregnancy and monitoring. Best practice & research. Clinical Obstetrics & Gynaecology. 2008;**22**(5):801-823

[10] Belfort M, Saade G, Foley M, Phelan J, Dildy G, editors. Critical Care Obstetrics. 5th ed. Singapore: Wiley-Blackwell; 2010

[11] Campbell JP, Bushby D, Yentis SM. Cardiopulmonary resuscitation in the pregnant patient: A manikin-based evaluation of methods for producing lateral tilt. Anaesthesia. 2013;**68**(7):694-699

[12] Gabbott DA. Uterine displacement during CPR in the pregnant patient-why bother? Resuscitation. 2013;**84**(3):267-268

[13] Ezri T, Lurie S, Weiniger CF, Golan A, Evron S. Cardiopulmonary resuscitation in the pregnant patient—An update. The Israel Medicine Association Journal. 2011;**13**(5):306-310

[14] Saenz-Madrigal ME, Vindas-Morera CA. Paro cardiaco en el embarazo. Revista Costarricense de Cardiología. 2013;**15**(2):1-9

[15] Dijkman A, Huisman CM, Smit M, et al. Cardiac arrest in pregnancy: Increasing use of perimortem caesarean section due to emergency skills training? British Journal of Obstetrics and Gynaecology. 2010;**117**:282

[16] Einav S, Kaufman N, Sela HY. Maternal cardiac arrest and perimortem caesarean delivery: Evidence or expert-based? Resuscitation. 2012;**83**:1191-1200. DOI: 10.1016/j. resuscitation.2012.05.005

[17] Katz V, Balderston K, DeFreest M. Perimortem cesarean delivery: Were our assumptions correct? American Journal of Obstetrics & Gynecology. 2005;**192**:1916-1920

[18] Lipman S, Daniels K, Cohen SE, Carvalho B. Labor room setting compared with the operating room for simulated perimortem cesarean delivery: A randomized controlled trial. Obstetrics & Gynecology. 2011;**118**:1090-1094. DOI: 10.1097/AOG.0b013e3182319a08

[19] Lipman S, Cohen S, Einav S, Jeejeebhoy F, Ahyre J, Morrison L, et al. The society for obstetric anesthesia and perinatology consensus statement on the management of cardiac arrest in pregnancy. Anesthesia & Analgesia.2014;**118**(5):1003-1016

[20] Perkins GD, Handley AJ, Raffay V, Monsieurs KG, Castren M. Resuscitation algorithms-linear or circular? Resuscitation. 2015;**88**:17-18

Chapter 4

Should Family be Allowed During Resuscitation

Abbas Al Mutair

Additional information is available at the end of the chapter

http://dx.doi.org/10.5772/intechopen.70189

Abstract

The practice of family presence during resuscitation provides the opportunity to the family members to attend visually and physically with the patient during resuscitation. The concept of family presence during resuscitation empowers the family-centred care philosophy. However, allowing families during resuscitation is controversial among health care providers. Using predefined search terms, a systematic search was carried out on CINAHL, PubMed, Proquest, Meditext, Ebsco and MedLine. Of the references identified, 35 studies were identified that met the inclusion criteria. The included studies clearly highlight. The family members revealed a desire to their presence during resuscitation and indicated further benefits of their presence. Health care providers had different opinions, some refused the practice indicating that it would be offensive and may interfere with the treatment. Others believed that it would positively affect patient care and would reassure family that the best care is being provided. Both family members and health care providers showed a need for educational programs and written policies to facilitate family presence during resuscitation.

Keywords: resuscitation, presence during resuscitation, family witnesses resuscitation, relatives, health professionals

1. Introduction

The idea of allowing family members to be present during resuscitation began at the Foote Hospital in Michigan in the United States of America in 1983 [1, 2]. This was when two family members refused to leave their loved one during resuscitation and asked to be with them even for few minutes to offer what they could during such a crisis event. The American Emergency Nurses Association in 1993 was the first professional organisation to develop evidence-based written guidelines endorsing the practice of family presence during resuscitation [3]. Over the years, the option for relatives to be present during resuscitation has been highly recommended by a number of medical organisations throughout the world.

Family presence during resuscitation is an important topic and of current debate among health care professionals. The literature has shown that attitudes of nurses, physicians and families towards family presence were found to be significantly different [4, 5]. Some health care providers feared that family members may end up having traumatic memories of the practice [6], whereas many family members indicated they would prefer to remain with the patient [4]. Physicians were found to be more against family presence during resuscitation than were nurses [7–9].

Many health care organisations, including the American Association of Critical-Care Nurses, American Heart Association, Emergency Nurses Association, Canadian Association of Critical Care Nurses, Royal College of Nursing, British Association for Accident and Emergency Medicine, European Federation of Critical Care Nursing Associations, European Society of Paediatric and Neonatal Intensive Care and European Society of Cardiology Council on Cardiovascular Nursing and Allied Professions have issued statements that family members of patients undergoing resuscitation should be given the option to remain during the procedure [3, 10–12].

2. Search strategy

An electronic comprehensive search of resulting references was conducted on CINAHL, PubMed, Proquest, Meditext, Ebsco and MedLine using the words 'family presence during resuscitation', 'health professionals', 'nurses' with 'family witnesses resuscitation', 'relatives' and 'resuscitation'. Articles were included only if the manuscript was published in a peer-reviewed journal and was based on an empirical study. The quality of the studies included in the review was appraised using Polit and Beck guide to critique research articles asking questions on the report of the research process to determine whether the findings are usable and of good quality [13]. Questions were on study purpose, research design, literature review, research question/hypothesis, study sample, data collection, study results and study recommendations (refer to **Table 1**).

Critique element	Questions to be asked
Study purpose	Is the purpose clear? Is it relevant to the practice? Will the study improve practice and add to the body of the knowledge?
Research design	Is there a framework/theory to guide the study? If there is no framework/theory, is it clear to identify? How the data were collected? Who will be studied? What is the plan for conducting the study?
Literature review	Is the literature review comprehensive? Is the literature review current? Are the majority of sources primary or secondary? Is the literature review well organised?
Research question/ hypothesis	Is the research question/hypothesis clearly stated? Does the question/hypothesis match the purpose of the study?
Study sample	How were the sample chosen? How large is the sample?
Data collection	What steps taken to collect data? How often data was collected and for how long? What instruments or tools were used? Is the tool valid and reliable? Were data analysis procedure appropriate?

Critique element	Questions to be asked
Study results	Is the research question/hypothesis answered? Were there limitations? Can generalisation be made? Are the results supported in the literature?
Study recommendations	Are recommendations for further use in practice? Is there identified need for further research? Can change be made in practice based on the results of the study?

Polit and Beck [13].

Table 1. Polit and Beck guide to critique research articles.

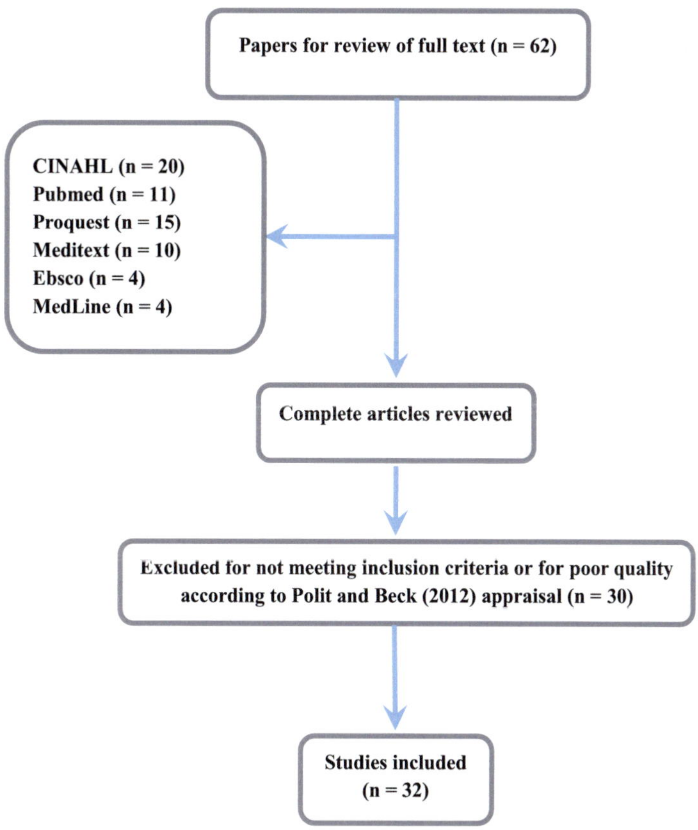

Figure 1. Literature review flow diagram.

As a result of the search, 62 articles were retrieved that were published between 1982 and 2016. These publications were mainly research reports, discussion and review papers. Most of the studies were descriptive and mainly used a quantitative approach to identify family presence during resuscitation and other invasive procedures [12, 14]. Fewer studies used an experimental design or qualitative approach. The majority of those studies were American in origin; however, some were Canadian, British, Swedish, Norwegian, Chinese, Icelandic, French, Australian, Turkish, Jordanian and German. In total, 32 English language publications were selected for this review. The excluded studies were either of poor quality or did not meet the inclusion criteria. This sample (n = 32) included seven papers that were published following the definition and initial development of family presence during resuscitation. A larger sample of 25 more recently published papers between 1990 and 2016 was included to represent the different perspectives of family presence during resuscitation (**Figure 1**). The attitudes of family members during resuscitation as perceived by family members will be discussed, followed by the attitude of health care providers towards the practice. However, before proceeding, the benefits of family presence during resuscitation are addressed.

3. Benefits of family presence

The benefits of family presence during resuscitation include several factors [7, 15, 16].

1. It assists in obtaining the patient's history quickly, thereby actively supporting the patient.
2. Family presence helps nurses to provide more holistic care.
3. Family presence encourages more professional behaviour among staff during resuscitation.
4. It strengthens the link between nurses and families and alleviates many of the doubts.
5. It provides an opportunity to educate the family about the condition of the patient.
6. The family presence during resuscitation and other invasive procedures reduces family anxiety and fear.
7. It is easier to manage family members when they are present in the room with the patient.
8. It enables family members to recognise that everything possible is being done to save the patient.
9. Family presence allows the opportunity for family members to say goodbye to their loved one when death occurs.

4. Family attitudes to family presence

The presence of family members during resuscitation can help them to face the reality of the situation and support the critically ill patient. Much of the literature has examined the attitudes of the family members towards their presence during resuscitation, but has neglected to explore the psychological effects of the practice on the family members.

In 1998, a small retrospective survey study took place at an inner-city teaching hospital in London [17]. The study was to assess the family members' desire to be present and to determine their knowledge of what was involved in the resuscitation process. Thirty-five family members who were not present during the resuscitation were asked to complete a questionnaire 3 months after their loved one's death. The findings suggested that only 4 (11%) of the 35 family members were given the option to be present during the resuscitation. Interestingly, of the total sample, 62% of family members would have chosen to be present during the resuscitation attempt if they had been given the option. This study indicated that most of the participating family members did not have an accurate idea of what occurred during the procedure. Therefore, their inclusion may have had a positive impact by knowing that everything possible was done to save their loved one. Family members of patients who survived were not included in the study and their inclusion would have added depth and enriched the study findings.

In the same year, Meyers et al. [18] completed a retrospective survey study of 25 family members who were not present during resuscitation, regarding their attitudes towards the practice. The participants were interviewed via telephone within 8 weeks to 15 months after the patient's death; all patients had received resuscitation and died within 1 h after admission to the hospital and 95% of the patients' deaths were caused by traumatic injury. The findings here revealed that 80% of family members who were surveyed indicated their desire to be with their loved one during resuscitation; 96% believed that they had the right to be present; 68% believed that their presence would have helped the patient and 64% felt their presence would have helped their sorrow following the death of their loved one. Regardless of the long period between the death of the family member and the data collection, the family members confirmed the benefit to the patient and family members and supported the option of being present [17, 18].

The third study which was a randomised controlled trial conducted in an Emergency Department (ED) in Cambridge, United Kingdom [15]. The study concerned the psychological effect on 18 family members who witnessed the resuscitation of their family member. The family members of patients who required resuscitation were divided into two groups: the first was the family members who were given the option to remain during the resuscitation ($n = 8$). The second was the family members who were not given the option to remain during the resuscitation ($n = 10$). The relatives were asked to complete five standardised psychological questionnaires within 1–6 months after the resuscitation. The small sample size and the criteria for subjects which were not provided in the article, have constrained the study findings. The findings showed that relatives who witnessed the resuscitation had lower levels of anxiety, intrusive imagery, depression and grief than did those who did not witness the resuscitation. No family members in the group reported being frightened or had to be asked to leave the room. The routine exclusion of family members from the resuscitation room may not be appropriate because family presence provides a means of expression for grieving family members.

Researchers using mixed methods surveyed family members to investigate their attitudes towards family presence during resuscitation and other invasive procedures [4]. They surveyed 39 family members, following 19 instances of family presence during resuscitation and 24 invasive procedures. The study indicated that all participating family members ascribed benefits in attending resuscitation. They added that for the families of dying patients, family presence afforded the opportunity to say goodbye and come to closure on a shared life for people who believed being with the patient was their right. Family members involved in resuscitation viewed themselves as 'active participants' in the care process, which met their needs for knowing about providing comfort and support for their loved one. All the participating family members surveyed in this study believed that visitation was helpful to them and noted that they would do it again. Also, almost all participants said they thought it was their right to be present with their loved one, and most importantly follow-up did not show they suffered from traumatic effects. They added that other benefits for the family included knowing that everything possible had been done, reducing their anxiety and fear and easing their bereavement. A strong bias can clearly be identified in the data collection, family members who accepted visitation during resuscitation or other invasive procedures were included in the study while those who refused it were excluded.

Differently from the previous studies, six family members whose loved ones underwent resuscitation and survived were interviewed within 24 h of the resuscitation [19]. This study was conducted in the Coronary Care Unit in a 700-bed urban community hospital in north eastern Ohio. The participants were adult family members and they were asked to describe the experiences, thoughts and perceptions of their critically ill relative during resuscitation in the ICU. The interviews showed that the family members were barred from the patients' room and asked to wait in another room. They struggled with the question of 'should we go or should we stay'. The author added that 'families lose autonomy and do not gain ground when they attempt to negotiate their way into the resuscitation room' (p. 417) [19]. The study concludes that when families are not provided information during resuscitation they cannot determine what is going on. Also, during the resuscitation of the loved one, the family is in crisis and needs reassurance and informational support to cope effectively. The study had a small sample size due to the exclusion of families whose relative underwent resuscitation and died. Although this exclusion criterion is understandable, it had influence on the power of the study as those members may have opinions and concerns to share that could have enriched to the study findings.

A randomised control trial design was used to study the attitudes of family members who were present during resuscitation [16]. The study was carried out by the researchers in a major tertiary referral teaching hospital in Queensland, Australia. Family members meeting the inclusion criteria were randomised to either the control group or experimental group. The control group (n = 40) did not attend the procedure and remained out of the resuscitation room. The experimental group (n = 58) were invited to the resuscitation room during resuscitation. A questionnaire was developed to gather the data for the study based on clinical staff experience and review of literature. The findings showed that the majority of family members in both the control and experimental group were grateful to be present during the resuscitation of their loved one. None of the participants felt pressured or traumatised to be present and 43% preferred to be present. Sixty-seven per cent of control group participants preferred to be present. Furthermore, in this study all of the family members who were present during resuscitation (experimental group) were glad that they were present to support their relative. The vast majority of the experimental group participants agreed that their presence during resuscitation helped them to come to terms with the patient's outcomes. Of the control group, 71.2% thought their presence would have helped them to cope better with their loved one's outcome. Participants in the experimental group (85%) felt their presence was beneficial to the patient's recovery. The findings of this research strongly support the presence of family during resuscitation, and have several clinical implications.

5. Healthcare providers' attitudes to family presence

The health care providers' behaviours towards family members often affect the family members' decision to be present or leave during the resuscitation. In 2000, three studies of health professional attitudes towards family presence during resuscitation were released using a survey design, which was conducted in three different contexts throughout the world. A retrospective study was conducted in a university-affiliated level I trauma centre [7]. The authors surveyed a total of 96 medical staff; 14 physicians, 22 residents and 60 nurses, who had participated in resuscitation or an invasive procedure with family members. The participants were asked to complete a 33-item questionnaire developed for the study within 17 days of the resuscitation or invasive procedure event.

Most of the medical staff (96% of nurses, 79% of physicians and 19% of the residents) favoured family presence during resuscitation. The vast majority (95% of the nurses, 77% of physicians and 64% of the residents) were comfortable with family presence during resuscitation. The study also evaluated the perceived stress of the 96 health care providers who had performed resuscitation efforts with family members present. The majority (84%) believed their performance was unaffected by the family's presence. The study concluded that the provider discomfort and inexperience decreased the likelihood of a supportive family presence. Also, the authors claim that family members should be assessed for their coping abilities and emotional stability before the option of family presence during resuscitation is offered. The study resulted in the development of a policy for family presence during resuscitation. The accuracy of the recollections of the medical staff may be questioned in Meyers et al.'s study [7], because the survey was completed over 2 weeks after the actual event.

In the second study, researchers surveyed 368 members of the American Association for the Surgery of Trauma (AAST) and 1261 Emergency Nurses Association (ENA) members [20]. The study proposed to determine the health care providers' opinion regarding the phase of the trauma resuscitation in which family members should be allowed to be present. The results indicated that only 3% of AAST members' participants, but 59% of ENA members, favoured family presence during resuscitation. The authors concede that the findings were biased by, firstly, the overrepresentation of ENA members, and secondly because the AAST members do not represent ED staff. Similarly to the previous study, the current study suggested the implementation of family presence may cause conflicts and thus impact on the performance of the trauma team [20].

In a third study a retrospective study was conducted in the Accident and Emergency (A&E) Department which took place at Hope Hospital Salford in the United Kingdom [21]. The study included only non-traumatic adult cardio pulmonary resuscitation and was to determine whether the presence of relatives during resuscitation altered perceived symptoms of stress in medical staff. An anonymous structured questionnaire was used to survey 114 medical staff 24 h after participating in resuscitation to obtain symptoms and acute stress reaction based on ICD-10 diagnostic criteria. The results indicated that 25 medical staff reported at least more than two symptoms of acute stress reaction. Of the 25 reporting more than two symptoms, 13 reported with the family being present during resuscitation and 12 without the family being present: there was thus no significant difference between the two groups. The study included only non-traumatic adult resuscitation and excluded the traumatic resuscitation which would have enriched the study findings. The findings here substantiate [7] findings that the presence of relatives witnessing resuscitation did not affect self-reported stress symptoms.

Researchers surveyed 592 health care professionals attending the International Meeting of the American College of Chest Physicians in San Francisco, using a quantitative method [8]. The questionnaire distributed consisted of six questions about family presence practice and resuscitation experience with relatives. The study found that fewer physicians (20%) compared to nurses and allied health care workers combined (39%), would allow family members presence during adult resuscitation. Thus study indicating that the majority of intensive care professionals did not support it. They added that the intensive care professionals' opposition was based on many reasons, which included the fear of psychological trauma to the witnessing family members, performance anxiety among the CPR team, and the distraction of the resuscitation team. However, others believed strongly that the presence of family members in the resuscitation bay would positively affect patient care. An interesting significant relationship of this study was found in that the health care professionals with previous experience of family presence opposed the practice more than those with no experience.

A quantitative descriptive research study was undertaken using a 30-item survey on a random sample of 1500 members of the American Association of Critical-Care Nurses and 1500 members of the ENA [9]. The study sought to identify policies, preferences and practices of critical care and emergency nurses towards family presence during resuscitation and invasive procedures. The survey consisted of 20 items on demographic data, 9 items on practice, preferences and policies and 1 item for comments and experiences of the nurse. A total of 473 intensive care nurses, 465 emergency nurses and 55 nurses who either practised in both areas or did not provide detailed work information participated in the study. The results indicate that nearly all of the 984 respondents had no written policies for family presence during resuscitation and other invasive procedures, and most preferred it to be allowed. Nearly half the participants indicated that they worked in units that allow family presence without written policies. Thirty-seven per cent of the respondents preferred written policies allowing family presence. Furthermore, most intensive care and emergency nurses supported the practice. These findings are consistent with [7] findings. The findings of this study also add to the evidence that health care providers who have experience with family presence tend to support the practice more than those who do not have experience, in contrast to Ref. [8].

These findings are important and have implications for conducting research on this issue in different settings because many nurses receive requests from patients' family members to be present during resuscitation and other invasive procedures and nurses are often the facilitators of the family presence. The study concluded that family presence during resuscitation lacked written policy. The study did not undergo reliability testing and appeared to have no construct validity, also the generalisability of the study is limited to nurses.

Ellison applied a descriptive correlational study with qualitative components to identify the relationship between demographic variables and nurses' attitudes and beliefs regarding family presence during resuscitation or invasive procedures [22]. These demographic variables included educational preparation, specialty certification, experience, completion of a family presence educational offering, age, sex and ethnicity. A total of 208 hospital nurses and New Jersey ENA members completed the questionnaire. The study found a statistically significant difference between positive attitudes towards family presence and higher educational preparation ($r = 0.216$, $P < 0.01$), certification in emergency nursing ($r = 0.216$, $P < 0.01$) and emergency nurse specialisation ($r = 0.234$, $P < 0.01$). These findings support [20] study that certified nurses had more favourable attitudes towards family presence than noncertified nurses.

Qualitative findings revealed that personal factors such as experience with crisis situations, ability to manage crisis situations and cultural differences between patients/families and nurses were identified as variables influencing respondents' attitudes towards family presence [22]. Qualitative findings also revealed organisational and social factors that can have a negative impact on nurses' attitudes towards family presence. Working in an environment with supportive colleagues such as those with higher education and specialised training was more likely to bring a change in behaviour. Additionally, nurses found family presence most acceptable when they or their families were patients [22]. Those findings are limited as the data was collected from only one hospital and one professional nursing organisation.

Another descriptive qualitative study was carried out [23]. The study explored nurses' beliefs regarding family presence during resuscitation. The data were gathered from ten Registered Nurses (RNs), one male and nine female with a minimum of 4 years clinical experience working in diverse acute care units through a semi structured interview. The interview consisted of 16 open-ended questions and lasted for 45 min. Certain findings in this study are similar to those in study [7], both studies revealed that families should be assigned with staff due to the possibility of psychological harm to the families; staff feelings of being watched; and increased professional behaviour on the part of the resuscitation team when families are present. The issue of disruption by family members was also raised but authors commented that nearly their entire health care provider sample of 60 RNs and 36 physicians responded that family behaviour towards resuscitation procedures was appropriate [7].

Findings in Refs. [9, 23] differed with respect to participants' views about the need for policies. Participants in Ref. [23] study were not asked to address the issue of having written policies regarding family presence. In contrast, findings from Ref. [9] indicated that most intensive care nurses preferred having policies in place for resuscitation. They also noted that nurses, more than physicians, supported family presence [9]. Family presence is not traditionally practised and it may not be considered, unless brought to the attention of administration by nursing staff committed to change their policy. The study group in current study was small ($n = 10$), the age group was limited to 31–41 years of age and those factors accordingly limited the generalisability of the study findings [23]. Furthermore, the setting of the interview was different for all nurses and this did not allow consistency in the interview process.

The experiences and attitudes of 124 European critical care nurses to the family presence during resuscitation of adult patients were explored [12]. The nurses were invited to participate in the study during the first conference of the European Federation of Critical Care Nursing

Associations which was held in Paris in May 2002. A self-administered questionnaire was used to capture the attitudes and experiences of nurses. It consisted of biographical data, 6 questions concerning nurses' experiences of the practice and 30 questions concerning nurses' attitudes of family presence during resuscitation. Generally, critical care nurses supported the presence of family members and the majority ($n = 94$, 76.4%) thought that allowing family members to be present would reassure them to see that everything possible was done to save the patient.

Further, a majority of the nurses ($n = 71$, 57.3%) believed that family might draw comfort from sharing the last moment with patient. Nurses from the UK, however, held significantly more positive attitudes towards the practice than their non-UK counterparts. A more important finding of this study was the strong agreement among nurses that there should be a member of the resuscitation team facilitating family members throughout the experience, including providing emotional support, explanations and interpretations of the procedure, to the attending families. The authors believed that cultural values varying from country to country in Europe may have affected the experiences and attitudes of nurses towards family presence during resuscitation. This study relied on convenience sampling of critical care nurses, so there are difficulties in generalising the results to other areas. Additionally, the questionnaire was based on a review of the existing literature rather than an already validated tool; thus its validity and reliability might be questioned. In spite of the study limitations, the authors propose that further policy be developed accordingly to guide clinical practice.

The concept of family presence during resuscitation has also been researched in the Turkish context [14]. This descriptive study with a quantitative approach sought to explore experiences and opinions of critical care nurses regarding family presence during resuscitation in Turkey. The data were gathered using a 43-item questionnaire [12, 14]. The questionnaire consisted of three main areas: demographic characteristics of nurses, experiences of family presence during resuscitation and nurses' opinions of family presence. The study took place at 10 hospitals, 4 affiliated with the Turkish MOH, 3 affiliated with universities and 3 affiliated with Social Security Agency hospitals. A total of 409 eligible critical care nurses returned the self-report questionnaire [14].

The results indicated that more than half of the nurses had no experience of family presence during resuscitation and none of them had ever invited family members to be present during resuscitation [14]. The study indicated that the majority of the nurses did not agree that it was necessary for family members to be with the patient during resuscitation and they did not want family members to be present. In fact, none of the Turkish hospitals that participated in this study had a protocol or policy allowing family members to be present during resuscitation. The findings reveal that critical care nurses in Turkey are not familiar with the concept of family presence during resuscitation; accordingly, the authors further recommended educational programs about this issue and policy changes within the hospitals to enhance critical care.

Researchers designed and implemented a program of family presence during resuscitation at the Urban Academic Medical Centre [24]. The study assessed the attitudes of all nurses and physicians regarding family presence during resuscitation, using a two group pre-test post-test design. The initial survey was completed by 86 nurses and 35 physicians and the follow-up survey was completed by 89 nurses and 14 physicians. The questionnaire included three parts, demographic information, professional attitudes and behaviours and personal and professional experience of the practice. Consistent with the study [7–9] found that nurses showed stronger support for the rights of patients to have their families present than did physicians on both surveys. The authors in this study failed to identify the psychological effects of family presence during resuscitation on medical staff; also a limitation that was highlighted by the authors was that anonymity of participants did not allow the authors to evaluate individual change in the practice. Despite the differing concerns of nurses and physicians, the implementation of a family presence program was successful and is now the standard practice at the hospital where the study was conducted.

At the same time that the study [24] was released, another study in different contexts has been published on family presence during resuscitation. It examined the perception of 90 emergency nurses towards the family presence during resuscitation at Cork University Hospital in Ireland [25]. The authors in this study used a descriptive quantitative design through a questionnaire utilised for the study, which was developed by the ENA. The sample was a convenience sample of 90 nurses working in a level 1 trauma ED with over 6 months' experience. The nurses were predominantly females (83.3%) in the 30–40 years age group and were employed as staff nurses (80%). Surprisingly, the study showed that 58.9% of the participants had invited family members to attend the resuscitation. Another 17.8% had not had the opportunity to do so, but would allow the family members to be present if the opportunity arose. However, 74.4% of the nurses preferred a written policy, which gives the family members the option of being present during resuscitation. In spite of using a quantitative design which did not allow the nurses' perceptions to be explored in detail, the study has clinical implications. The study emphasised the need to develop educational programs for nurses on the safe implementation and practices of families witnessing resuscitations.

A descriptive study using survey methods was conducted to investigate the outcomes of family presence on staff attitude immediately post-resuscitation [26]. The findings here are part of a larger project of family presence that was conducted at a tertiary referral hospital in Brisbane in Queensland, Australia. The participants of this study were any medical staff members present during resuscitation of patients who met the inclusion criteria for the study. The inclusion criteria for an eligible resuscitation were Australian patients presenting as Triage Categories 1 or 2, with or without an altered level of consciousness, hypotension, respiratory distress or the need for CPR. The majority of the informants were nurses, followed by registrars, residents, consultants then social workers. In this survey, the staff felt there were positive aspects and advantages for relatives being present during resuscitation. These advantages include being able to obtain a medical history quickly; the patients being comforted by having relatives present; and the relatives benefiting by being present; thus the staff thought it was easier to manage while the relatives were present.

This study provided an Australian and international perspective to the existing research literature on staff attitudes to family members present during resuscitation, and a new perspective as well by examining staff attitudes immediately post-resuscitation. The findings of this study further support the presence during resuscitation within an environment that supports staff to undertake the care of the patients with their family being present.

Nurses' opinions of family presence during resuscitation have been influenced by culture and religion, according to Cunes [27]. This study [12, 14] replicated survey to determine the experiences and attitudes of Turkish intensive care nurses concerning family presence during resuscitation. Using a descriptive design research study, they surveyed 135 intensive care nurses from 2 university hospitals in Izmir by structured questionnaires [12, 27]. The vast majority (88.1%) disagreed that family members should be given the option to remain with their loved one during resuscitation. Only 22.2% of the intensive care nurses participated in resuscitation where family members were present. Almost all nurses (91.1%) agreed that they did not want family members to be present.

In addition, all nurses indicated that they had no protocol on family presence during resuscitation. Nurses agreed (72.6%) that family members, if present, would interfere with the resuscitation team performance and 86.6% of nurses believed that witnessing resuscitation by family members is a traumatic experience and a very stressful situation. The findings of this study are consistent with those of Ref. [14] as to the lack of support of Turkish intensive care nurses, which is a result of nurses having no knowledge, and neither policy nor protocol for family presence during resuscitation. The researchers concluded that educational programs, if implemented together with the developmental of protocols and guidelines, should both aid in the acceptance of the concept by the intensive care nurses in Turkey. The instrument used did not have any open-ended questions to allow nurses to write their additional thoughts.

Authors from Germany conducted another descriptive survey study to explore the German intensive care nurses' experiences and attitudes towards family presence during resuscitation [28]. The study used the questionnaire which was developed by Fulbrook et al. [12]; however, a fourth section was added to allow delegates to further write any additional concerns related to the issue. Unlike Ref. [12], this qualitative data enhanced both the depth and comprehensiveness of the participants' experiences. A total of 164 intensive care nurses were recruited who attended the 26th Reutlinger Fortbildungstage held in Reutlingen, Baden-Wurttemberg, Germany during September 2008. According to the researchers, most of the participants (68%) did not agree that family members should be given the option of being present during the resuscitation of their loved one. Also, over half (56%) were concerned that family presence would disturb the performance of the resuscitation team.

Consistent with Ref. [12] informants in this study, 73.5% agreed that there should be a dedicated member of the resuscitation team who should be available to meet the family needs, for instance to support and explain the resuscitation procedure to the family members. Moreover, 68% of nurses believed that family presence could help them to know that everything possible was done for their patient, which was also found [12]. Nurses in this study indicated that they rarely invited family to be present, which might be due to the lack of unit protocol or practice guideline. Researchers interpreted that the nurses' decision regarding practice might have been influenced by the German cultural values and societal traditions. The study encouraged simulation training techniques to assist practitioners to increase their confidence, overcome their fears and support the family during the situation: those topics are to be introduced within the nursing curricula.

In Iran, a study was undertaken to determine the opinions of health care providers of family presence during resuscitation and other invasive procedures in four teaching hospitals in

Tehran [29]. A total of 200 health care providers were surveyed by a questionnaire developed for the study which asked about the demographic characteristics of the respondents, years of working experience and opinions about relatives' presence during intubation and resuscitation. The participants' age, gender, experience and speciality did not correlate with the participants' attitudes towards family presence. However, participants with previous exposure to family presence were more in favour of family presence. Similar to a study previously sampled from nurses in another Muslim community in Turkey [14], the results of this study revealed that the majority (77.9%) opposed the practice. The most common reasons for the participants' opposition, as indicated by the authors, were the health care providers' fear of psychological trauma to family members, possible interference with patient care as the Muslim families are potentially closer and more prone to display emotions which may distract the resuscitation team.

Further, a total of 132 nurses were surveyed nurses using a self-administered questionnaire in two hospitals in Saudi Arabia [30]. The study found that 75.6% of the participants did not support the family presence practice indicating the same reasons as Ref. [29] for opposition such as witnessing resuscitation is a traumatic experience and fearing that family members will negatively impact on the resuscitation team. An interesting finding was a statistically significant relationship between nurses with previous experience of family presence and support for the practice [30]. Nurses with previous experience of family presence opposed the practice more than nurses with no previous experience ($P = 0.001$). However, this was not the case where ICU health care providers with previous experience of family presence during resuscitation were found to be more supportive of the practice, compared to the health care providers with no previous experience [28]. Authors maintained that the Islamic religion and the Saudi culture influenced the nurses' attitudes towards the practice of family presence [30].

Significantly, different perceptions can be perceived regarding family presence during resuscitation [31]. However, studies have shown that family members consider the need to be close to the patient as very important as the unpredicted admission without any warning causes high level of stress and anxiety among family members [31]. Additionally, the experience resuscitation creates an intense emotional situation for both patients and their family members [32]. The health care providers reported a need for training programmes to support the family when they attend resuscitation [30–32]. A number of studies also emphasised the need to develop educational programmes for medical staff on the safe implementation and practice of family presence [12, 24, 28]. The health care providers also indicated the need to develop policies to support family involvement and give family the option to attend resuscitation [31].

6. Conclusion

In general, most of the reviewed studies were descriptive, using either quantitative or qualitative approaches. The family members in those earlier reviewed studies indicated their desire and supported their presence during resuscitation. They also advocated further benefits including helping the patient, knowing everything possible was done to save their loved one and support provided to grieving family members. These findings highlight the importance of giving the health care providers the confidence in including the family during the care of the patient and considering them as part of the caring team. The studies also demonstrated that health care providers have significantly different opinions regarding family presence during resuscitation. Some oppose family presence for many reasons including that the practice would be offensive, produces stress in staff and that family members may interfere with the treatment. Other health care providers were comfortable with the family presence and believed that it would positively affect patient care, agreeing that their presence would reassure them that the best care is being provided. It was obvious that the research so far has failed to identify the psychological effects of family presence on the families during resuscitation. Regardless of the difference in health care providers' views, some endorsed the need for written policies to allow family presence and others suggested a 'nurse facilitator' dedicated to evaluate readiness of the family members to attend the procedure and explain it to them when they attend.

The findings of this research suggest a number of recommendations, including clinical implications and further research which include the following:

6.1. Clinical implication

The decision to implement the family presence practice should be well prepared. The decision needs to be made at the individual level (health care providers) and organisational level (hospitals). The study helped also to identify some issues which needed to be addressed before offering the option to families to be present during the resuscitation attempts on their family member. The identified issues include guidelines, written policies, informed consent and family presence educational programs.

A significant concern should be given to the family presence policy. The policy must ensure providing the family members a safe and caring environment. Before the option is offered, the families should be assessed for coping abilities and the absence of extreme psychological and emotional disturbance. The policy also should stress on the nurse facilitator interventions regarding the follow-up and explanations to the family throughout the procedure. Therefore, this study suggested a proposed practice standard (Appendix A) that could help to fulfil the family as a whole, rather than treating the patient individually and assures the safe implementation of family presence during the resuscitation of the loved one.

Secondly, the family presence educational programs should benefit the health care providers and families who would like to attend the resuscitation of their loved one. Accordingly, staff support programs should be developed to assist families who want to be present during resuscitation. Health care facilities also should contribute educational sessions on the family presence practice for the society to be well informed and have adequate knowledge of the practice. Through different teaching strategies, the family presence practice can be instructed to the participants such as lectures or pamphlets. This study suggested a proposed assessment of the family members to cope with the situation, and the infection control practices for safe implementation by the health care providers.

6.2. Further research

Future studies should include other health care providers' attitudes regarding family presence practice. It is most important to study the view of patients and family members as to whether they really want to and benefit from being the family presence during resuscitation for both adults and paediatric patients. This study also will act as a stimulus for further research in an area of family presence during resuscitation.

6.3. Recommendations for successful family presence program

- Development of protocol of family presence practice.
- Attendance at educational program regarding family presence for all staff involved in the practice.
- Program should include:
  - Assessment of family members' ability to cope with the situation and the absence of extreme emotional disturbance behaviours.
  - Removal of the non-essential equipment from the resuscitation room in order to make space for the family members.
  - Infection control practices, for example, the family members may be asked to wear gloves, gown or eye protection to prevent exposure to blood or body fluids.

7. Standard of practice for family presence during resuscitation

7.1. Definition

It is the presence of family members during the resuscitation of their loved one.

7.2. Purpose

To treat the patients and families holistically and to support the family needs.

7.3. Policy statement

Family members will be permitted in the patient care during resuscitation of their family member.

7.4. Procedure

1. The nurses will be responsible for assessing patient and family needs to be present during resuscitation.

2. The facilitator nurse is responsible for assessing the family members' ability to cope with the situation and the absence of extreme emotional disturbance behaviours before the option can be offered.
3. If the facilitator nurse agrees to allow the family members during the resuscitation, the patient (if conscious) will be asked if they agree for the family to be present.
4. Only two of family members will be allowed in the resuscitation room, prioritising the next of kin and at this time the consent must be secured by the family members.
5. Prior to entering the resuscitation room, the facilitator will explain to the relatives about the patient's condition, treatments and equipment available in the room, where they stand in the room and when they may leave if any psychological distress appears.
6. The family members will be accompanied by the facilitator in the resuscitation room.

The nurse facilitator will:

- Explain the procedure to the family members.
- Provide information about the expected outcomes and the patient's response to the treatment.
- Reassure the relatives, open space for the family's point of view and answer their questions.

Author details

Abbas Al Mutair

Address all correspondence to: abbas4080@hotmail.com

Inaya Medical College, Riyadh, Saudi Arabia

References

[1] Doyle CJ, Post H, Burney RE, Maino J, Keefe M, Rhee KJ. Family participation during resuscitation: An option. Annuls of Emergency Medicine. 1987;**16**:673-675

[2] Hanson C, Strawser D. Family presence during cardiopulmonary resuscitation: Foote Hospital emergency department's nine-year perspective. Journal of Emergency Nursing. 1992;**18**:104-106

[3] Emergency Nurses Association. Family presence at the bedside during invasive procedures and cardiopulmonary resuscitation. Emergency Nurses Association White Paper. 2005:1-6

[4] Meyers TA, Eichborn DJ, Guzzetta CE, Clark AP, Taliaferro E. Family presence during invasive procedures and resuscitation: The experience of family members, nurses, and physicians. Topics in Emergency Medicine. 2004;**26**(1):61-73

[5] Moreland P, Manor B. Family presence during invasive procedures and resuscitation in the emergency department: A review of the literature. Journal of Emergency Nursing. 2005;**31**(1):58-72

[6] Redley B, Hood K. Staff attitudes towards family presence during resuscitation. Accident & Emergency Nursing. 1997;**4**;145-151

[7] Meyers T, Echhorn D, Guzzetta C, Clark C, Klein J, Taliaferro, E. Family presence during invasive procedures and resuscitation: The experience of family members, nurses, and physicians. Advanced Emergency Nursing Journal. 2000;**31**(1):58-72

[8] McClenathan B, Torrington K, Uyehara C. Family member presence during cardio-pulmonary resuscitation: A survey of US and international critical care professionals. American College of Chest Physicians. 2002;**122**(6):2204-2211

[9] Maclean S, Guzzetta C, White C, Fontaine D, Eichhorn D, Meyers T, Desy P. Family presence during cardiopulmonary resuscitation and invasive procedures: Practices of critical care and emergency nurses. American Journal of Critical Care. 2003;**12**(3):246-257

[10] American Heart Association. Guidelines 2000 for cardiopulmonary resuscitation: Part 2. Ethical Aspects of CPR and ECC. 2000;**102**:112-121

[11] Canadian Association of Critical Care Nurses. Family Presence During Resuscitation. 2006. Retrieved from: http://www.caccn.ca/

[12] Fulbrook P, Albarran J, Latour, J. A European survey of critical care nurses' attitudes and experiences of having family members present during cardiopulmonary resuscitation. International Journal of Nursing Studies. 2005;**42**:557-568

[13] Polit D, Beck C. Nursing Research: Generating and Assessing Evidence for Nursing Practice. 9th ed. Philadelphia: Lippincott Williams & Wilkins; 2012

[14] Badir A, Sepit D. Family presence during CPR: A study of the experiences and opinions of Turkish critical care nurses. International Journal of Nursing Studies. 2007;**44**(20):83-92

[15] Robinson S, MacKenzie-Ross S, Campbell G, Egleston C, Prevost A. Psychological effect of witnessed resuscitation on bereaved relatives. The Lancet. 1998;**352**:614-617

[16] Holzhauser K, Finucane J, Vries S. Family presence during resuscitation: A randomised controlled trial of the impact of family presence. Australasian Emergency Nursing Journal. 2006;**8**:139-147

[17] Barratt F, Wallis N. Relatives in the resuscitation room: Their point of view. Journal of Accident Emergency Medicine. 1998;**15**:109-111

[18] Meyers A, Echhorn J, Guzzetta CE. Do families want to be present during CPR? A retrospective survey. Journal of Emergency Nursing. 1998;**24**:400-405

[19] Wanger J, Kent A, Ohio K, Ohio C. Lived experience of critically ill patients' family members during cardiopulmonary resuscitation. American Journal of Critical Care. 2004;**13**(5):416-420

[20] Helmer D, Shapiro M, Dors M, Karan S. Family presence during trauma resuscitation: A survey of American Association of Sleep Technologists and Emergency Nurses Association members. Journal of Trauma Injury Infection Critical Care. 2000;**48**:1015-1020

[21] Boyd R, White S. Does witnessed cardiopulmonary resuscitation alter perceived stress in accident and emergency staff? European Journal of Emergency Medicine. 2000;**7**:51-53

[22] Ellison S. Nurses' attitudes toward family presence during resuscitative efforts and invasive procedures, Journal of Emergency Nursing. 2003;**29**(6):515-521

[23] Knott A, Kee C. Nurses' beliefs about family presence during resuscitation. Applied Nursing Research. 2005;**18**;192-198

[24] Mian P, Warchal S, Whitney S, Fitzmaurice J, Tancredi K. Impact of a multifaceted intervention on nurses' and physicians' attitudes and behaviours toward family presence during resuscitation. Critical Care Nurse. 2007;**27**(1):52-61

[25] Madden E, Condon C. Emergency nurses current practices and understanding of family presence during CPR. Journal of Emergency Nursing.2007;**33**(5):433-440

[26] Holzhauser K, Finucane J. Part B: A survey of the staff attitudes immediately post-resuscitation to family presence during resuscitation. Australasian Emergency Nursing Journal. 2008;**11**:114-122

[27] Cunes U, Zaybak A. A study of Turkish critical care nurses' perspectives regarding family-witnessed resuscitation. Journal of Clinical Nursing. 2009;**18**:2907-2915

[28] Koberich S, Kaltwasser A, Rothaug O, Albarran J. Family witnessed resuscitation—Experience and attitudes of German intensive care nurses. British Association of Critical Care Nurses. 2010;**5**(15):241-250

[29] Kianmeher N, Mofidi M, Rahmani H, Shahin Y. The attitudes of team members towards family presence during hospital-based CPR: A study based in the Muslim setting of four Iranian teaching hospitals. Journal of Royal College and Physicians of Edinburgh. 2010;**40**:4-8

[30] Al-Mutair A, Plummer V, Copnell B. Family presence during resuscitation: A descriptive study of nurses' attitudes from two Saudi hospitals. Nursing in Critical Care. 2012;**17**(2):90-98

[31] Al-Mutair AS, Plummer V, O'brien A, Clerehan R. Family needs and involvement in the intensive care unit: A literature review. Journal of Clinical Nursing. 2013;**22**(13-14): 1805-1817

[32] Mohamed Z, Sasikala M, Nurfarieza MA, Ho SE. Needs of family members of critically ill patients in a Critical Care Unit at Universiti Kebangsaan Malaysia Medical Centre. Medicine & Health. 2016; **11**(1):11-21

Section 3

Extending Guidelines and Research

Chapter 5

Chest Compression-Only Cardiopulmonary Resuscitation

Hui-Chun Chen and Shoa-Lin Lin

Additional information is available at the end of the chapter

http://dx.doi.org/10.5772/intechopen.70830

Abstract

The survival rate of out-of-cardiac arrest (OHCA) was very low, which was mainly due to the victims who do not receive cardiopulmonary resuscitation (CPR) immediately. It was estimated that if people who quickly get chest compression-only CPR while awaiting medical treatment have double or even triple the chance of surviving. In the true world, many individuals are unwilling to do mouth-to-mouth breathing due to fear of infections or unable to do mouth-to-mouth breathing at the same time in the situation of only one bystander. This article has performed an extensive review in order to update the concept of chest compression-only CPR.

Keywords: cardiac arrest, cardiopulmonary resuscitation (CPR), chest compression, out-of-hospital cardiac arrest (OHCA), return of spontaneous circulation (ROSC)

1. Introduction

More than 300,000 Americans died from cardiac arrest each year [1]. Cardiopulmonary resuscitation (CPR) provided by a bystander may improve outcome [2] but is generally performed in less than 30% of the cases [3, 4].

Survival rate of out-of-cardiac arrest (OHCA) is only about 7% [5] in previous 2 decades. According to etiology, cardiac arrest can be divided into asphyxial and non-asphyxial types. Asphyxial arrest is caused by situations inducing low blood oxygen status, like drawing, suicide on the hanging, monoxide carbon intoxication, etc. The non-asphyxial arrest is due to dysfunction of cardiac electrical activity [6]. This article will focus in non-asphyxial OHCA patients. The major reason of low survival rate of OHCA patients is that they do not receive CPR immediately. The 2010 American Heart Association (AHA) guidelines made a change of the sequence of CPR from A, airway; B, breathing; C, chest compression (A-B-C) to C-A-B to put an emphasis on chest compression and its rate and depth. This change could make CPR more easy to start and minimize delaying time for ventilation. Starting CPR from mouth-to-mouth ventilation is a big barrier in real world due to fear of communicating infectious disease or other reasons. Except that it is easier to start CPR from chest compressions, this change from A-B-C to C-A-B make the cardiac arrest patient earlier to receive chest compression which is the most important element of CPR. The delay time for ventilation would also be shorter than before, like receiving ventilation after 30 chest compressions or is about only 18 seconds of delay at the speed of at least 100 chest compression/minute or even shorter if there two bystanders who resuscitated children or infant. Chest compression-only CPR is encouraged in certain condition like only one rescuer, untrained rescuers, or multiple rescuers who are unwilling to do mouth-to-mouth ventilation [7]. There are randomized trials that support results of chest compression-only CPR recently [8, 9]. Chest compression-only CPR is easier to do by untrained bystander and is easier to be introduced by dispatcher by phone and increase actual provision by bystanders [10].

In this work, we will firstly describe our recent successful experience treating a case with OHCA after chest compression-only CPR who has complete neurological recovery [11] and perform an extensive review in order to update the concept of chest compression-only CPR.

2. Case presentation

A 55-year-old male had smoking history for 40 years but without prior history of diabetes mellitus, hypertension, or hyperlipidemia. He developed collapse suddenly in the presence of his exercise partners when playing tennis. One exercise partner called for emergency medical service (EMS) team, and another partner began chest compression-only CPR immediately. The compression-only CPR was performed by one bystander for the initial 8 minutes, followed by two persons alternatively. After 28 minutes, the paramedic team arrived. At that time, the patient was unresponsive, no detectable blood pressure, pulseless, and without spontaneous respiration. The EMS team secured the airway and performed ventilation via Ambu bagging and continuous chest compression. After 10 minutes of CPR, the EMS found a detectable carotid pulse, the ECG monitor showed sinus rhythm but with wide QRS complex. For the prehospital resuscitation, the return of spontaneous circulation (ROSC) was achieved after 28 minutes of chest compression-only CPR by bystanders plus 10 minutes of assisted ventilation/chest compression by EMS. The patient had a blood pressure of 180/105 mmHg, heart rate of 88/minute, respiratory rate of 12/minute, and SpO2 of 99%. Nevertheless, he was still unresponsive with Glasgow Coma Scale of E1V1M1. The patient was then transported to our emergency department where he received endotracheal intubation immediately. The vital signs revealed body temperature, 36.1°C; pulse rate, 125 bpm; respiratory rate, 20/minute; blood pressure, and 122/96 mmHg, but the coma scale was E1V1M1. He was transferred to the intensive care unit promptly. His conscious level mildly improved from E1V1M1 to E2VTM3 after admitted at the intensive care unit. On the third admission day, his consciousness recovered (from E2VTM3 to E4V5M6), and he was extubated. He was transferred to the general ward on the fourth hospital day. On the fifth hospital day, the percutaneous coronary intervention and electrophysiological study were suggested, but patient refused due to a personal reason. A computed tomographic coronary angiogram studied on the sixth hospital day showed significant stenosis of the right coronary artery and heavy calcifications of both left anterior and left circumflex coronary arteries. On the seventh hospital day, he was discharged without any neurological or memory impairment. Thus, this case supports the present CPR guideline that recommends effective chest compression without assisted ventilation by laypersons for managing patients in cardiac arrest.

3. Searching strategy

We use a medical term as "chest compassion-only CPR" and search relevant papers from the PubMed, Medline + Journals@ Ovid, and Cochrane library. There were no restrictions for sex or populations. We do not restrict search criteria to humans or animals. We only limit search criteria to English language, review articles, and publication year from January 2010 to August 2017. We limit that the publication year is hoping to get the most updated information. We found that there were 35 review articles from PubMed, 11 review articles in Medline + Journals@ Ovid, and 1 review article in Cochrane, respectively. The repeated data were found in 10 articles; thus, only 37 articles were obtained in the systemic review. We will report the updated information relevant to the chest compression-only CPR. Other issues including mechanical chest compression devices, pharmacological agents in cardiac arrest, and post-resuscitation care are not included in this article.

4. Increasing rates of bystander CPR

Successful treatment of OHCA patients remains an unmet health demand. The crucial components of treatment consist of early recognition of cardiac arrest, prompt and effective CPR, effective and early defibrillation, and organized post-resuscitation care. The initiation of bystander CPR followed by a prompt emergency response delivers high-quality CPR, which is critical to patients' outcomes. Before 2010, most OHCA patients do not receive any bystander CPR even if there is a bystander at the scene [12]. One of the probable reasons is due to the A-B-C sequence of CPR, which makes rescuers feel difficult to start CPR from opening the airway and delivering breaths with mouth-to-mouth ventilation. The bystanders would rather call emergent medical service (EMS) team and await emergency staff to arrive to start CPR. Thus, such cardiac arrest patient's outcome is very poor. Bystanders do not start CPR because they are afraid of get hurt, contacting infectious disease, not enough confidence to practice complicated conventional CPR, and following legal problems [13]. Changing CPR sequence as C-A-B in 2010 AHA guideline might encourage rescuers more easily to begin CPR from starting with chest compressions compared with staring from mouth-to-mouth ventilation. Besides, this change can let OHCA patients receive chest compression earlier without delay due to giving ventilation. Giving ventilation first not only delays chest compression but also increases thoracic pressure, decreases venous return, and decreases coronary artery pressure. This vicious cycle brings poor prognosis of cardiac arrest victim. A recent report found that the chance of selecting compression-only CPR markedly increased from 36.4% in 2005–2007 to 63.7% in 2011–2012 [14]. This change in results may be explained by the increase of dispatcher instruction to lay rescuers, concept change after the 2010 AHA guideline, and most importantly the dissemination of compression-only CPR in the CPR training program [15, 16]. Thus, a few recommendations may be helpful to increase rate of bystander CPR including to broaden CPR training, provide reassurance to increase participation, improve EMS quality which are discussed in this section.

4.1. Broaden CPR training

In order to spread and accelerate CPR education, new approaches are required to reach a larger public audience. Lynch et al. have develop and validate a 30-minute CPR self-instruction program for laypersons [17]. This CPR course has provided a useful tool for education outside the classroom. Another way to broaden CPR training might be through recently developed automated external defibrillator (AED) programs. The Cardiac Arrest Survival Act (CASA; Public Law 106–505) mandated establishment of lay rescuer AED programs in federal buildings. Many state governments have carried out AED programs in public places, like airport, hotels, gymnasiums, schools, nursing homes, and train stations. CPR trainings held by governments are inspired to provide CPR training for future rescuers as part of the comprehensive community lay rescuer AED plans. The AHA has provided information to schools to help them prepare to respond to medical emergencies, including sudden cardiac death [18].

4.2. Dispatcher-assisted "telephone CPR"

The broadened CPR training is helpful to the public laypersons. However, these CPR trainings may not resolve the problem for the cardiac arrest victims that occur at home, where only a few untrained witnesses may commonly be present. The development of dispatcher-assisted "telephone CPR" may allow for CPR instruction in real time even when rescuers have not received prior training. Dispatcher-assisted "telephone CPR" is especially important for cardiac arrest at home where without trained rescuers or available AEDs. Dispatcher-assisted CPR instruction variations have been surveyed [19, 20] and have found that this "training" method was a useful technique to lay rescuers for direct CPR care.

4.3. Offer reassurance to increase participation

Bystander reluctance to perform CPR is common. The government officers must announce that the chance of disease transmission is very low. To the best of our knowledge, there was no case report of human immunodeficiency virus or hepatitis transmission through performance of CPR up-to-date. In combination with Occupational Safety and Health Administration recommendations for places of working, decision-makers should provide devices of mouth-to-mouth barrier and gloves where AEDs are available. Those devices can assist CPR performance when AEDs are used. CPR classes should be included in Good Samaritan legislation [21] and published near AED installations. The public should realize that the survival chance of OHCA victim can be double or triple if bystanders practicing CPR immediately, while the CPR performance is at little risk to the rescuer.

4.4. Strengthen CPR practice and EMS quality

Lay rescuers and EMS training projects of the community must include a course of continuous quality improvement that includes reviewing of resuscitation attempts, CPR quality, and dispatcher CPR instructions that will be offered to bystanders. Healthcare provider systems must perform continuous quality improvement plans that include monitoring the quality of CPR practiced during any resuscitation efforts. These monitored data must be used to maximize resuscitation care quality, including CPR practice quality. Nowadays, several devices have been made to both estimate and offer feedback about CPR practice, either extra capabilities of CPR monitor of defibrillators or stand-alone equipment which rescuers can use before a defibrillator available at the scene of cardiac arrest [22, 23]. Some of these devices, like "piston-type mechanical cardiopulmonary resuscitation device," can also record CPR performance and provide opportunities for training [24]. These tools may have an important impact on this quality improvement goal.

5. Quality of chest compression element of CPR

Chest compression is the most important element of CPR. Excellent chest compression can maximize coronary perfusion pressure and increase the chance of ROSC. Chest compression helps blood from the heart to arterial system and coronary artery system. At the release phase of chest compression, the blood returns to the heart under negative thoracic pressure, so that external chest compression helps the "heart works again" and provides about 30% blood supply as normal heart works [25, 26].

New data continuously come out which validate the importance of both the practicing CPR *per set* and assuring CPR quality are most favorable. The International Liaison Committee for Resuscitation performed a systematic review of evidence for the optimal chest compression characteristics during the 2010 Consensus on Science and Treatment Recommendations Conference. The final conclusions of this review were recommendations for deeper (≧5 cm) and quicker (≧100/minute) chest compressions, ensuring full release of pressure between compression and minimizing interruptions in chest compressions [27]. Here we will discuss in-depth of each element of CPR.

5.1. Chest compression rate and depth

External chest compression rate is suggested at least 100/minute in 2010 AHA guideline. Chest compression number is an important determination of survival with good neurological function and ROSC which is the most powerful predictor of survival from OHCA [3]. The OHCA patient who receives chest compression rate between 100 and 120/minute has a greatest chance to survival to discharge according to 2010 AHA guideline [28].

Except chest compression rate, chest compression depth is suggested to at least 2 in (5 cm) in 2010 AHA guideline but not 1½–2 in (4–5 cm) before. Chest compression depth directly compresses the heart and increases to create intrathoracic pressure to generate blood flow, which bring oxygen to the brain and heart. Deeper chest compression is associated with higher chance of survival to hospital. Every 0.5 cm increase depth doubles the chance of successful resuscitation [29]. Enough depth of chest compression is also a key to survival. However, chest compression depth has a reverse relation to chest compression rate. The higher chest compression rate and the lower chest compression depth have been noted. If chest compression rate up to 145/minute is done, the depth of chest compression becomes unacceptable according to 2005 AHA guideline [30].

The 2010 AHA guideline suggests chest compression depth of at least 2 in (5 cm) in adult's CPR equally without consideration of patients' thoracic diameter and body size. If chest compression depth is too deeper (residual of chest diameter less than 2 cm), chest compression may not be helpful to patient but hurt intrathoracic organs and lead to complications. For low-body-weight patients, an alternative chest compression depth of one-fourth of the external anterior to posterior thoracic depth is recommended [31].

5.2. Allowing complete chest recoil

Not only emphasizing chest compression rate and depth, but allowing total chest complete recoil at each chest compression is also mentioned by 2010 AHA guideline. Complete chest recoil makes negative thoracic pressure to draw venous blood back to the heart and thus increases preload of the heart, higher coronary perfusion pressure, and good cerebral perfusion pressure. Allowing complete chest recoil at each chest compression is suggested at the speed of at least 100 chest compressions/minute. But this condition will make rescuer easily fatigue because upward force needs to be full against gravity which induce major energy consumption of the rescuer. Fatigue of rescuer will lead to chest wall incomplete decompression and smaller chest compression depth and increase residual intrathoracic pressure during chest decompression stage. Increased residual intrathoracic pressure will obscure venous return, make less increase in systemic arterial pressure when chest compression, and decrease cerebral and coronary perfusion pressure. Even 1 minute of incomplete chest decompression during CPR will bring negative effect [32]. Changing sequential persons is an effective way to keep cardiopulmonary resuscitation quality by keeping chest compression rate at least 100/minute and allowing complete chest recoil.

5.3. Minimalize chest compression interruptions

Minimalizing chest compression interruptions is an index of high quality of chest compression component. Chest compression phase replaces systolic pressure of the heart, and the recoil phase replaces diastolic pressure of the heart. Chest compression interruptions result in no cardiac support during CPR. This situation is called no flow time (NFT). Such chest compression interruptions make poor prognosis of OHCA [33, 34]. The change of the ventilation to chest compression ratio from 2:15 to 2:30 according to 2005 CPR guideline suggests to increase chest compression velocity per minute and minimalize interruptions induced by ventilation. These interruptions made 25% reduction in the NFT [35].

Chest compression is also interrupted by pulse and rhythm check. Cessation of chest compression for automated external defibrillators (AEDs) to analyze electrocardiogram can lead to 10% no flow time (NFT) events. When asystole and ventricular fibrillation (VF) are analyzed, additional confirmatory pulse checking makes delay chest compression. These two kinds of no flow times (NFTs) can be prevented by immediate chest compression when asystole is revealed by electrocardiogram or just defibrillated ventricular fibrillation (VF) rhythm. Filtering out artifact wave from chest compression by cardiac monitor or automated external defibrillator (AED) avoids chest compression interruptions and increases cardiopulmonary resuscitation (CPR) efficiency [36].

Pre-/post-defibrillation pauses may cause chest compression interruptions and create no flow times (NFTs) due to defibrillator charging, pulse and rhythm check, or lack of quick chest compressions [37]. Shortening pre-/post-defibrillation pauses of chest compression increases 13-fold chance of ROSC [38]. Besides, decrease pre-defibrillation pause of chest compression increases chance of successful defibrillation and effects of termination ventricular tachycardia (VT)/ventricular fibrillation (VF) situation [39]. Even now, a safe and effective tool for "hands-on" defibrillation solves chest compression interruption of pre-/post-defibrillation pause and increases chance of successful defibrillation. Though, it is still studied [40].

In out-of-hospital cardiac arrest (OHCA), transferring patient from arrest situation to ambulance is also a reason of no flow time (NFT) [41]. Rescuers should be educated that transferring cardiac arrest patient can lead to NFT. Besides, rescuer team should not move OHCA patient until ROSC is successful after giving professional advance life resuscitation or move OHCA patient with compressions and using Advance Cardiology Consultants and Diagnostics (ACCDs) [42].

Besides, many other reasons can influence the chest compression interruptions. Cardiopulmonary resuscitation scene has a high emotional stress; human behavior can cause nonspecific NFTs. Like poor leadership, poor task distribution by a leader who gives double or even triple orders which lead rescuer hard to member to produce high cognition load will result in poor rescuer concentration and poor awareness of CPR situations. The abovementions will cause nonspecific NFTs. In the contrast, if the leader gives rescuer members a single, clear order which can make rescuers decrease cognition load increases teamwork quality and decreases NFTs [43]. There are several common reasons causing NFTs [43], such as (1) rescuer fatigue and change chest compressor, (2) performing ventilation, (3) performing airway maintenance, (4) application CPR device, (5) pulse and rhythm check, (6) pre-/post-defibrillation pause, (7) performing vascular access, and (8) transferring patient to ambulance.

Rescuer fatigue and change chest compressor are the most common reasons to induce NFT events. Especially, chest compressor fatigue is usually found after 1 minute of CPR work. In 2010 AHA guideline, chest compressor change every 2 minutes is suggested. Changing chest compressors also interrupts chest compression. To minimize chest compression interruptions, chest compressor switch must be done within 5 seconds. If there are two rescuers, they should be positioned on either side of the patient. One rescuer should be ready and wait to change "working compressor" every 2 minutes [44].

5.4. Avoid excessive ventilation

In 2010 AHA guideline, rescue ventilation is less emphasized than before. During low blood flow due to cardiopulmonary resuscitation status, oxygen supply is mainly from limited blood flow, and chest compression presents as "working heart." Thus, chest compression is emphasized in the first few minutes of witnessed cardiac arrest [45]. Excessive ventilation increases high thoracic pressure which results in lower coronary perfusion pressure, decreased venous return, and poor survival rate [46]. In 2010 AHA guideline, suggested ventilator rate during CPR is giving two breaths (1 second each) during a brief (about 3–4 seconds) pause after is every 30 chest compressions [47].

In conclusion, chest compression is the key component of CPR. High quality of chest compression is the mostly important determination of ROSC which is the most important predictor of survival from cardiac arrest. Besides, high quality of chest compression combined by rate and depth, minimalizing chest interruptions, and avoiding excessive ventilation, is an important determination of survival with good neurological outcome [3].

6. Compression-only CPR

Compression-only CPR is easier to teach; it does not require mouth-to-mouth ventilation (which can be an impediment to bystanders starting CPR), and it reduces interruptions in chest compressions. Hupfl et al. [8] have conducted a systematic review and meta-analysis in two settings of CPR in OHCA patients—chest compression-only bystander CPR and standard bystander CPR (chest compression plus rescue ventilation). A primary meta-analysis included trials that patients of those trials were randomized to attribute to accept one of the two CPR techniques which are commended by dispatchers, and another meta-analysis included studies of chest compression-only CPR as observational cohort studies. Survival to hospital discharge was the primary outcome. The pooled data of three randomized trials revealed that chest compression-only CPR survival chance was greater (14% [211/1500]) than that of the standard CPR (12% [178/1531]; risk ratio 1.22, 95% CI 1.01–1.46). The absolute increase in survival was 2.4% (95% CI 0.1–4.9). In the secondary meta-analysis of seven observational cohort studies, no difference was recorded between the two CPR techniques (8% [223/2731] and 8% [863/11152]; risk ratio 0.96, 95% CI 0.83–1.11). They concluded that for adults with out-of-hospital cardiac arrest, instructions to bystanders from emergency medical services dispatch should focus on chest compression-only CPR.

A more recent review reported by Zhan et al. [6] have compared the effects of continuous chest compression CPR (with or without rescue breathing) versus conventional CPR plus rescue breathing (interrupted chest compression with pauses for breaths) of non-asphyxial OHCA in large scales of patients. They included three randomized controlled trials (RCTs) and one cluster RCT (with a total of 26,742 participants analyzed). According to CPR methods, this report divided CPR into "CPR administered by untrained bystander" and "CPR administered by a trained professional."

For the *CPR administered by untrained bystander*, bystanders administered CPR under telephone instruction from emergency services. They found that better OHCA patient survival to hospital discharge rate (2.4%; 14 versus 11.6%; RR 1.21, 95% confidence interval (CI) 1.01–1.46; 3 studies, 3031 participants) was those who received continuous chest compression CPR without rescue breathing compared with those who received interrupted chest compression with rescue breathing (ratio 15:2). For the *CPR administered by a trained professional* from emergency medical service (EMS) professionals, there were 23,711 participants who received either continuous chest compression CPR (100/minute) with asynchronous rescue breathing (10/minute) or interrupted chest compression with pauses for rescue breathing (ratio 30:2). Results revealed that lower risk of survival to hospital discharge was noted for continuous chest compression CPR with asynchronous rescue breathing (9.0%) compared with interrupted chest compression with rescue breathing (9.7%). Both have an adjusted risk difference (ARD) of −0.7%; 95% CI (−1.5 to 0.1%) (moderate-quality evidence).

Return of spontaneous circulation is likely to be slightly lower in people treated with continuous chest compression CPR plus asynchronous rescue breathing (24.2 versus 25.3%; −1.1% (95% CI −2.4 to 0.1)) (high-quality evidence).

This report found that following OHCA, bystander-administered chest compression-only CPR, supported by telephone instruction, increases the proportion of people who survive to hospital discharge compared with conventional interrupted chest compression CPR plus rescue breathing. However, when CPR performed by EMS providers, continuous chest compressions plus asynchronous rescue breathing did not result in higher rates for survival to hospital discharge compared to interrupted chest compression plus rescue breathing [6]. Thus, due to these experiences, it is reasonable to suggest that bystander should perform CPR and as soon as possible (1) do basic life support protocol, if trained (in CPR) and willing and (2) do compression-only CPR, if untrained or unwilling to include ventilation. Healthcare professionals should perform CPR with combined compressions and ventilations.

Another animal study compared survival of VF-arrested swine treated with chest compression-only CPR or with realistic bystander CPR where each set of chest compressions was interrupted with a realistic 16 seconds for ventilations. Survival was 80% with chest compression-only CPR and 13% with standard bystander CPR [18]. Similar authors have performed their extensive efforts to advocate and teach chest compression-only CPR as part of cardiocerebral resuscitation for patients with primary cardiac arrest in the state of Arizona. They found that for OHCA patients, the survival rate was 7.8% in those receiving guidelines of CPR and 13.3% for those who received chest compression-only CPR. In the subset of patients with a witnessed cardiac arrest and a shockable rhythm, the survival rate was 17.7% in those receiving guidelines of CPR and 34% in those patients receiving chest compression-only CPR [49, 50]. These findings support the usefulness of chest compression-only CPR in managing OHCA patients.

7. Future direction

It has been reported that the use of Internet-based CPR education and certification may expand current training program coverage, according to the expanding use of Internet via television, mobile telephone, and other personal devices [51]. In certain conditions, simpler procedure of by bystander resuscitation, like chest compression-only CPR, may broaden participation and remain a field that needs further studies [20]. For EMS-CPR and resuscitation companies, college or institute of EMT training systems, and other professional CPR providers, the use of accurate simulation with video recording and debriefing may be very useful in resuscitation training; the use of such patient simulators is rapidly an expanding area that deserves a lot of attention [52, 53].

8. Conclusion

OHCA remains a common event and is associated with high mortality. Strengthening the chain of survival with prompt initiation of high-quality CPR, minimizing interruptions in chest compressions and organized post-resuscitation care, provides focused opportunities to improve outcomes. CPR must be started as soon as possible after a victim of OHCA, and bystander should (1) do full CPR, if trained (in CPR) and willing and (2) do chest compression-only CPR, if untrained or unwilling to perform mouth-to-month ventilation. Healthcare professionals should perform CPR with combined compressions and ventilations. Improved survival rates depend on a public trained and motivated to recognize the emergency, activate EMS or the emergency response system, initiate high-quality CPR, and use an AED if available.

Author details

Hui-Chun Chen[1] and Shoa-Lin Lin[2,3]*

*Address all correspondence to: sllin@yuanhosp.com.tw

1 Department of Internal Medicine, Kaohsiung Municipal Min-Sheng Hospital, Kaohsiung City, Taiwan

2 Division of Cardiology, Department of Internal Medicine, Yuan's General Hospital, Kaohsiung City, Taiwan

3 National Defense Medical College, Taipei, Taiwan

References

[1] Lloyd-Jones D, Adams R, Carnethon M, et al., American Heart Association Statistics Committee and Stroke Statistics Subcommittee. Heart disease and stroke statistics: 2009 update: A report from the American Heart Association Statistics Committee and Stroke Statistics Subcommittee. Circulation. 2009;**119**(3):480-486

[2] ECC Committee, Subcommittees and Task Forces of the American Heart Association. 2005 American Heart Association Guidelines for cardiopulmonary resuscitation and emergency cardiovascular care. Circulation. 2005;**112**(24 Suppl):IV1-IV203

[3] Sasson C, Rogers MA, Dahl J, Kellermann AL. Predictors of survival from out-of-hospital cardiac arrest: A systematic review and meta-analysis. Circulation: Cardiovascular Quality and Outcomes. 2010;**3**(1):63-81

[4] Nichol G, Thomas E, Callaway CW, et al., Resuscitation Outcomes Consortium Investigators. Regional variation in out-of-hospital cardiac arrest incidence and outcome. Journal of the American Medical Association. 2008;**300**(12):1423-1431

[5] Berdowski J, Berg RA, Tijssen JG, Koster TW. Global incidences of out-of-hospital cardiac arrest and survival rates: Systematic review of 67 prospective studies. Resuscitation. 2010;**81**(11):1479-1487

[6] Zhan L, Yang LJ, Huang Y, He Q, Liu GJ. Continuous chest compression versus interrupted chest compression for cardiopulmonary resuscitation of non-asphyxial out-of-hospital cardiac arrest. Cochrane Database of Systematic Reviews. March 27, 2017;**3**: CD010134

[7] Field JM, Hazinski MF, Sayre MR, et al. Part 1: Executive summary: 2010 American Heart Association Guidelines for cardiopulmonary resuscitation and emergency cardiovascular care. Circulation. 2010;**122**(18 Suppl 3):S640-S656

[8] Hupfl M, Selig HF, Nagele P. Chest-compression-only versus standard cardiopulmonary resuscitation: A meta-analysis. Lancet. 2010;**376**:1552-1557

[9] Zhan L, Yang LJ, Huang Y, He Q, Liu GJ. Continuous chest compression versus interrupted chest compression for cardiopulmonary resuscitation of non-asphyxial out-of-hospital cardiac arrest. Cochrane Database of Systematic Reviews. 2017;**3**:CD010134

[10] Shimamoto T, Iwami T, Kitamura T, et al. Dispatcher instruction of chest compression-only CPR increases actual provision of bystander CPR. Resuscitation. 2015;**96**:9-15

[11] Chen HC, Hung YM, Hsieh FC, Lin SL. A case of neurologically intact survival after compression-only cardiopulmonary resuscitation by two bystanders. Hong Kong Journal of Emergency Medicine. 2016;**23**:371-375

[12] Fujie K, Nakata Y, Yasuda S, Mizutani T, Hashimoto K. Do dispatcher instructions facilitate bystander-initiated cardiopulmonary resuscitation and improve outcomes in patients with out-of-hospital cardiac arrest? A comparison of family and non-family bystanders. Resuscitation. 2014;**85**(3):315-319. DOI: 10.1016/j.resuscitation.2013.11.013 Epub 2013 Nov 26

[13] Bobrow BJ, Panczyk M, Subido C. Dispatch-assisted cardiopulmonary resuscitation: The anchor link in the chain of survival. Current Opinion in Critical Care. 2012;**18**(3):228-233

[14] Fukuda T, Ohashi-Fukuda N, Kobayashi H, et al. Conventional versus compression-only versus no-bystander cardiopulmonary resuscitation for pediatric out-of-hospital cardiac arrest. Circulation. 2016;**134**(25):2060-2070

[15] Iwami T, Kitamura T, Kiyohara K, Kawamura T. Dissemination of chest compression-only cardiopulmonary resuscitation and survival after out-of-hospital cardiac arrest. Circulation. 2015;**132**:415-422

[16] Goto Y, Maeda T, Goto Y. Impact of dispatcher-assisted bystander cardiopulmonary resuscitation on neurological outcomes in children with out-of-hospital cardiac arrests: A prospective, nationwide, population-based cohort study. Journal of the American Heart Association. 2014;**3**:e000499. DOI: 10.1161/JAHA.113.000499

[17] Lynch B, Einspruch EL, Nichol G, Becker LB, Aufderheide TP, Idris A. Effectiveness of a 30-min CPR self-instruction program for lay responders: A controlled randomized study. Resuscitation. 2005;**67**:31-43

[18] Hazinski MF, Markenson D, Neish S, et al., American Heart Association; American Academy of Pediatrics; American College of Emergency Physicians; American National Red Cross; National Association of School Nurses; National Association of State EMS Directors; National Association of EMS Physicians; National Associations of Emergency Medical Technicians; Program for School Preparedness and Planning; National Center for Disaster Preparedness; Columbia University Mailman School of Public Health. Response to cardiac arrest and selected life-threatening medical emergencies: The medical emergency response plan for schools: A statement for healthcare providers, policymakers, school administrators, and community leaders. Circulation. 2004;**109**:278-291

[19] Hallstrom AP, Cobb LA, Johnson E, Copass MK. Dispatcher assisted CPR: Implementation and potential benefit: A 12-year study. Resuscitation. 2003;**57**:123-129

[20] Dias JA, Brown TB, Saini D, et al. Simplified dispatch-assisted CPR instructions outperform standard protocol. Resuscitation. 2007;**72**:108-114

[21] The Good Samaritan Law across Europe, from: http://www.daneurope.org/c/document_library/get_file?uuid=c09228f3-a745-480b-9549-d9fc8bbbd535&groupId=10103, accessed on August 3, 2017

[22] Kramer-Johansen J, Myklebust H, Wik L, et al. Quality of out-of-hospital cardiopulmonary resuscitation with real time automated feedback: A prospective interventional study. Resuscitation. 2006;**71**:283-292

[23] Abella BS, Edelson DP, Kim S, et al. CPR quality improvement during in-hospital cardiac arrest using a real-time audiovisual feedback system. Resuscitation. 2007;**73**:54-61

[24] Huang EP, Wang HC, Ko PC. Obstacles delaying the prompt deployment of piston-type mechanical cardiopulmonary resuscitation devices during emergency department resuscitation: A video-recording and time-motion study. Resuscitation. September 2013;**84**(9): 1208-1213

[25] Barsan WG, Levy RC. Experimental design for study of cardiopulmonary resuscitation in dogs. Annals of Emergency Medicine. 1981;**10**(3):135-137

[26] Jiang L, Zhang JS. Mechanical cardiopulmonary resuscitation for patients with cardiac arrest. World Journal of Emergency Medicine. 2011;**2**(3):165-168

[27] Koster RW, Sayre MR, Botha M, et al. Part 5: Adult basic life support: 2010 International consensus on cardiopulmonary resuscitation and emergency cardiovascular care science with treatment recommendations. Resuscitation. 2010;**81**(Suppl 1):e48-e70

[28] Idris AH, Guffey D, Pepe PE, et al. Chest compression rates and survival following out-of-hospital cardiac arrest. Critical Care Medicine. 2015;**43**(4):840-848

[29] van Alem AP, Vrenken RH, de Vos R, Tijssen JG, Koster RW. Use of automated external defibrillator by first responders in out of hospital cardiac arrest: Prospective controlled trial. British Medical Journal, 2003;**327**:1312

[30] Edelson DP, Abella BS, Kramer-Johansen J, et al. Effects of compression depth and pre-shock pauses predict defibrillation failure during cardiac arrest. Resuscitation. 2006;**71**(2): 137-145

[31] Lee SH, Kim DH, Kang TS, et al. The uniform chest compression depth of 50 mm or greater recommended by current guidelines is not appropriate for all adults. American Journal of Emergency Medicine. 2015;**33**(8):1037-1041

[32] Yannopoulos D, SMcKnite S, Aufderheide TP, et al. Effects of incomplete chest wall decompression during cardiopulmonary resuscitation on coronary and cerebral perfusion pressures in a porcine model of cardiac arrest. Resuscitation. 2005;**64**(3):363-372

[33] Wik L, Kramer-Johansen J, Myklebust H, et al. Quality of cardiopulmonary resuscitation during out-of-hospital cardiac arrest. Journal of the American Medical Association. 2005;**293**(3):299-304

[34] Valenzuela TD, Kern KB, Clark LL, et al. Interruptions of chest compressions during emergency medical systems resuscitation. Circulation. 2005;**112**(9):1259-1265

[35] Hostler D, Rittenberger JC, Roth R, et al. Increased chest compression to ventilation ratio improves delivery of CPR. Resuscitation. 2007;**74**:446-452

[36] Berger RD, Palazzolo J, Halperi H. Rhythm discrimination during uninterrupted CPR using motion artifact reduction system. Resuscitation. 2007;**75**(1):145-152

[37] Caparon MH, Rust KJ, Hunter AK, et al. Integrated solution to purification challenges in the manufacture of a soluble recombinant protein in *E. coli*. Biotechnology & Bioengineering. 2010;**105**(2):239-249

[38] Sell RE, Sarno R, Lawrence B, et al. Minimizing pre- and post-defibrillation pauses increases the likelihood of return of spontaneous circulation (ROSC). Resuscitation. 2010;**81**(7):822-825

[39] Olsen JA, Brunborg C, Steinberg M, et al. Pre-shock chest compression pause effects on termination of ventricular fibrillation/tachycardia and return of organized rhythm within mechanical and manual cardiopulmonary resuscitation. Resuscitation. 2015;**93**:158-163

[40] Yu T, Ristagno G, Li Y, Bisera J, Weil MH, Tang W. The resuscitation blanket: A useful tool for "hands-on" defibrillation. Resuscitation. 2010;**81**(2):230-235

[41] Krarup NH, Terkelsen CJ, Johnsen SP, et al. Quality of cardiopulmonary resuscitation in out-of-hospital cardiac arrest is hampered by interruptions in chest compressions – A nationwide prospective feasibility study. Resuscitation. 2011;**82**(3):263-269

[42] Souchtchenko SS, Benner JP, Allen JL, Brady WJ. A review of chest compression interruptions during out-of-hospital cardiac arrest and strategies for the future. Journal of Emergency Medicine. 2013;**45**(3):458-466

[43] Fernandez Castelao E, Russo SG, Cremer S, et al. Positive impact of crisis resource management training on no-flow time and team member verbalisations during simulated cardiopulmonary resuscitation: A randomised controlled trial. Resuscitation. 2011;**82**(10): 1338-1343

[44] Berg RA, Hemphill R, Abella BS, et al. Part 5: Adult basic life support: 2010 American Heart Association Guidelines for cardiopulmonary resuscitation and emergency cardiovascular care. Circulation. 2010;**122**(18 Suppl 3):S685-S705

[45] Chandra NC, Gruben KG, Tsitlik JE, et al. Observations of ventilation during resuscitation in a canine model. Circulation. 1994;**90**(6):3070-3075

[46] Aufderheide TP, Sigurdsson G, Pirrallo RG, et al. Hyperventilation-induced hypotension during cardiopulmonary resuscitation. Circulation. 2004;**109**(16):1960-1965

[47] Neumar RW, Otto CW, Link MS, et al. Part 8: Adult advanced cardiovascular life support: 2010 American Heart Association Guidelines for cardiopulmonary resuscitation and emergency cardiovascular care. Circulation. 2010;**122**(18 Suppl 3):S729-S767

[48] Ewy GA. Chest compression only cardiopulmonary resuscitation for primary cardiac arrest. Circulation. 2016;**134**:695-697

[49] Bobrow BJ, Clark LL, Ewy GA, et al. Minimally interrupted cardiac resuscitation by emergency medical services for out-of-hospital cardiac arrest. Journal of the American Medical Association. 2008;**299**:1158-1165. DOI: 10.1001/jama.299.10.1158

[50] Ewy GA. Cardiocerebral resuscitation: The new cardiopulmonary resuscitation. Circulation. 2005;**111**:2134-2142

[51] Choa M-H, Park I-C, Chung HS, Yoon YS, Kim S-H, Yoo SK. Internet-based animation for instruction in cardiopulmonary resuscitation. Journal of Telemedicine and Telecare. 2006;**12**(Suppl 3):31-33

[52] Marsch SC, Tschan F, Semmer N, Spychiger M, Breuer M, Hunziker PR. Unnecessary interruptions of cardiac massage during simulated cardiac arrests. European Journal of Anaesthesiology. 2005;**22**:831-833

[53] Wayne DB, Butter J, Siddall VJ, et al. Mastery learning of advanced cardiac life support skills by internal medicine residents using simulation technology and deliberate practice. Journal of General Internal Medicine. 2006;**21**:251-256

Chapter 6

Audiovisual Feedback Devices for Chest Compression Quality during CPR

Digna M. González-Otero, Sofía Ruiz de Gauna,
Jesus M. Ruiz, José Julio Gutiérrez,
Purificación Saiz and Mikel Leturiondo

Additional information is available at the end of the chapter

http://dx.doi.org/10.5772/intechopen.70742

Abstract

During cardiopulmonary resuscitation (CPR), chest compression quality is the key for patient survival. However, several studies have shown that both professionals and laypeople often apply CPR at improper rates and depths. The use of real-time feedback devices increases adherence to CPR quality guidelines. This chapter explores new alternatives to provide feedback on the quality of chest compressions during CPR. First, we describe and evaluate three methods to compute chest compression depth and rate using exclusively the chest acceleration. To evaluate the accuracy of the methods, we used episodes of simulated cardiac arrest acquired in a manikin model. One of the methods, based on the spectral analysis of the acceleration, was particularly accurate in a wide range of conditions. Then, we assessed the feasibility of using the transthoracic impedance (TI) signal acquired through defibrillation pads to provide feedback on chest compression depth and rate. For that purpose, we retrospectively analyzed three databases of out-of-hospital cardiac arrest episodes. When a wide variety of patients and rescuers were included, TI could not be used to reliably estimate the compression depth. However, compression rate could be accurately estimated. Development of simpler methods to provide feedback on CPR quality could contribute to the widespread of these devices.

Keywords: cardiopulmonary resuscitation, chest compression quality, compression depth, compression rate, feedback devices, chest acceleration, thoracic impedance

1. Introduction

The sequence of actions linking a victim of out-of-hospital cardiac arrest with survival is described by the chain of survival, which consists of four independent links: early activation of the emergency medical services, early cardiopulmonary resuscitation (CPR), early defibrillation, and early advanced care. The four links of the chain of survival are important, but early CPR and early defibrillation are pivotal for a successful outcome of the patient [1]. CPR consists of cycles of chest compressions and ventilations delivered to the patient to artificially maintain a minimal flow of oxygenated blood to the vital organs, whereas defibrillation consists in the passage of electrical current through the myocardium (cardiac muscle) to terminate certain lethal arrhythmias. In out-of-hospital settings, early defibrillation is normally procured using an automated external defibrillator (AED).

There is a strong evidence that the quality of chest compressions is related to the chance of successful defibrillation [2–4]. Current resuscitation guidelines [1] emphasize the importance of providing chest compressions with an adequate depth (between 5 and 6 cm) and rate (between 100 and 120 compressions per minute [cpm]), completely releasing the chest between compressions and minimizing interruptions. However, several studies have shown that both professionals and laypeople often apply CPR at improper rates and depths [5, 6].

In an effort to alleviate this problem, since 2010, resuscitation guidelines recommend monitoring CPR quality and using metronomes and real-time feedback systems to guide rescuers during resuscitation attempts [7]. Metronomes generate regular audible beats that help rescuers to follow the rhythm, while feedback devices are more sophisticated; they measure CPR performance in real time and provide audiovisual messages to guide the rescuer toward target depth and rate. The clinical studies conducted to date had an insufficient power to demonstrate improved survival with the use of feedback devices [8]. As a consequence, ERC guidelines 2015 recommend the use of CPR feedback devices as part of a broader system of care that should include comprehensive CPR quality improvement initiatives, rather than as an isolated intervention. There is, however, strong evidence that feedback improves chest compression quality, [9–12] which has been linked to survival from cardiac arrest [5, 8].

This chapter explores new alternatives to provide feedback on the quality of chest compressions during CPR. First, we briefly describe the history of feedback devices and the different technologies used. Then, we present three methods to provide feedback on chest compression depth and rate based solely on chest acceleration. One of the methods presented particularly a high accuracy in a wide range of conditions and is further discussed in three challenging scenarios. Finally, we assessed the feasibility of using the transthoracic impedance (TI) signal acquired through defibrillation pads to provide feedback on chest compression depth and rate.

2. History of feedback devices

The first CPR feedback devices were mechanical and used force or pressure sensors to provide feedback on chest compression depth [13]. Devices in this category include CPRplus (Kelly Medical Products, Princeton, USA), CPREzy (Health Affairs, London, England), and the more recent Cardio First Angel (Schiller, Baar, Switzerland). These systems guide the rescuer toward the target depth based on the force applied on the chest for each compression. However, stiffness of the chest is not linear [14] and varies among individuals. Tomlinson et al. [15]

http://dx.doi.org/10.5772/intechopen.70742

simultaneously measured compression force and depth in 91 adult out-of-hospital cardiac arrest patients. In the studied population, the force required to achieve 38 mm varied from 10 to 54 kg. Even if some of the devices in this category take into account the approximate size of the patient, the wide variation in chest wall elasticity and its changes with time impede an accurate estimation of compression depth from compression force.

To overcome the limitations of force and pressure sensors, electronic systems based on accelerometers were developed. These devices sense the acceleration of the patient's chest during CPR, and they process it in real time to obtain compression depth. By definition, acceleration is the first derivative of velocity with respect to time, and velocity is the first derivative of displacement. Consequently, chest displacement can be obtained from acceleration by applying double integration. However, integration is an inherently unstable process: small integration errors rapidly accumulate causing a significant drift in displacement that impedes accurate estimation of the compression depth. **Figure 1** illustrates the problem of double integration of the chest acceleration with a record acquired while chest compressions were provided to a resuscitation manikin. The acceleration signal (top panel) and the reference compression depth signal obtained from a displacement sensor placed inside the manikin's chest (bottom panel, solid line) were registered. The second panel shows the reference velocity signal computed differentiating the reference compression depth signal (solid line), and the velocity signal computed by numerically integrating the acceleration signal (dashed line). Integration errors quickly accumulate, and during the last seconds, the computed velocity presents a noticeable offset with respect to the reference signal. When numeric integration is performed again, this offset leads to big errors in the computed displacement (bottom panel, dashed line), of more than 20 cm after only 8 s in this example.

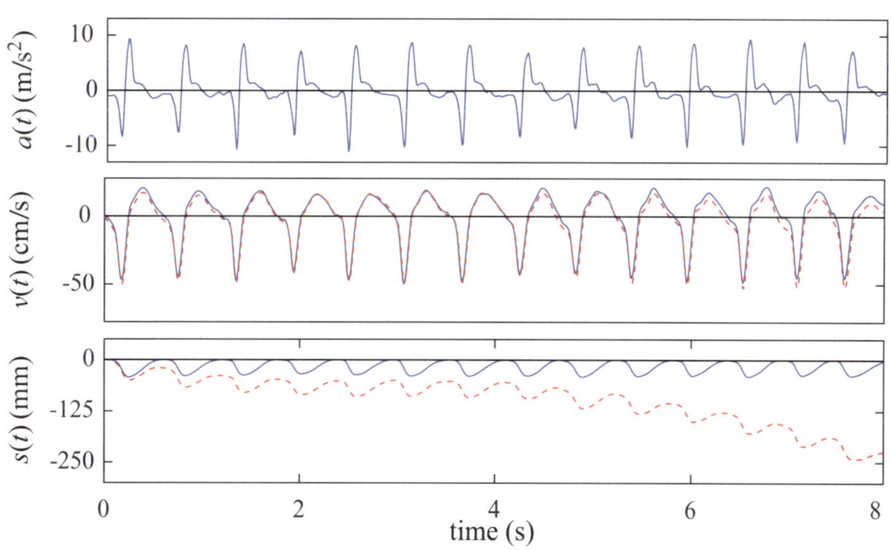

Figure 1. Integration errors in the displacement signal after the application of direct double integration to the acceleration signal.

A possible strategy to reduce the accumulation of integration errors would be to perform the integration for small signal segments, for example, for each compression cycle. For that purpose, the offset of each chest compression should be first identified, and the integration should be reset by applying boundary conditions after each cycle, that is, setting velocity and displacement at those points to zero. Over the last decade, several mechanisms to identify the offset of chest compressions have been conceived, giving rise to complex commercial devices that incorporate additional sensors or use elaborate signal processing techniques. For example, PocketCPR (Zoll Medical, Chelmsford, USA) applies signal processing techniques to set boundary conditions and compensate integrating drift, while CPRmeter (Laerdal Medical, Stavanger, Norway) incorporates an additional force sensor. Both devices are rigid and must be placed between the chest of the patient and the rescuer's hands during CPR to measure chest acceleration.

More recently, Physio-Control (Redmond, USA) presented TrueCPR, a solution to provide feedback on chest compression rate, depth, and chest release based on triaxial magnetic field induction. The device comprises two rigid pads: one of them is positioned between the rescuer's hands and the chest of the patient during CPR, and the other one, longer and flatter, beneath the patient's back. Feedback metrics are estimated from the changes in magnetic field between both pads during CPR. The main disadvantage of this device is that it is bulkier than the others and also rigid.

3. Use of the acceleration signal for chest compression quality

This section briefly describes three methods to compute chest compression rate and depth and to provide CPR feedback to the rescuers using only chest acceleration. For a more detailed description of the methods, see reference [16]. The first method derives from the traditional approach; it consists in applying double integration to compute the compression depth signal. In our proposal, integration is approximated using a stable band-pass filter (BPF) that performs integration while suppressing low frequencies of the signal. The second and third methods do not require computing the compression depth signal: the second method computes velocity to calculate a compression rate and depth value for each compression, while the third one computes rate and depth from the spectral analysis of the acceleration signal (SAA). We used episodes of simulated cardiac arrest acquired using a resuscitation manikin to evaluate the accuracy of the three methods.

3.1. Experimental set-up and data collection

We equipped a Resusci Anne QCPR manikin (Laerdal Medical, Norway) with a photoelectric sensor to register the reference compression depth signal. Chest compressions were delivered in the center of the manikin's chest with a triaxial accelerometer encased in a metal box placed beneath the rescuer's hands. The reference compression depth signal and the three axes of the acceleration were digitized and recorded using a National Instruments (Austin, USA) acquisition card connected to a laptop computer. **Figure 2** shows the experimental set-up used to perform the data collection.

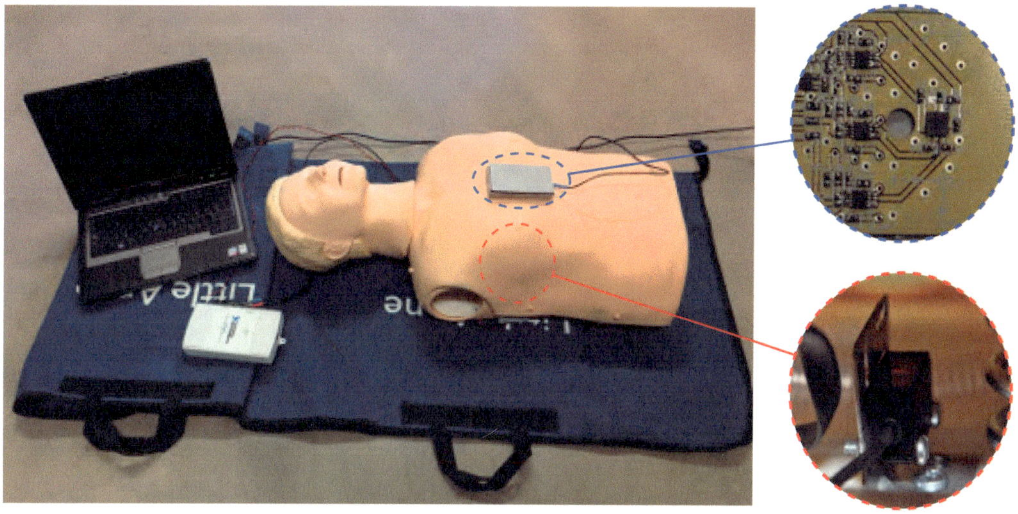

Figure 2. Experimental setup: Resusci Anne QCPR manikin fitted with a displacement sensor, triaxial accelerometer encased in a metallic box, acquisition card, and laptop computer.

Twenty-eight volunteers participated in the recording sessions. They were grouped in couples, and for each couple, four 10-min episodes were recorded. During each episode, volunteers alternated providing 2-min CPR series, each series involving 30 compressions with 5-s pauses in between. A total of 56 episodes were acquired. The experimental protocol was approved by the ethical committee for research involving human subjects of the University of the Basque Country (CEISH UPV/EHU).

3.2. Methods to estimate chest compression rate and depth

3.2.1. Band-pass filter

There are a number of discrete integration algorithms available, the most common one being the trapezoidal rule, because of its trade-off between simplicity and accuracy. Analytically, the implementation of this rule derives in an unstable linear system [16]. In practice, that means that small low-frequency components in the input signal generate low-frequency components in the output with amplitude that increases with time. If no technique is applied to compensate this accumulation of error in the output signal, the system could suffer a numeric overflow.

Our first approach consists in approximating the integration by a stable band-pass filter, designed as the series connection of a high-pass filter and the trapezoidal rule filter, which presents a low-pass response. The high-pass filter is aimed at compensating the instability of the trapezoidal rule filter for low frequencies. **Figure 3** shows the magnitude of the frequency response of the band-pass filter, $H_{BPF}(f)$, represented by a solid line. Note that for frequencies above 0.6 Hz, the system matches the ideal response of the trapezoidal rule, depicted with a dashed line, whereas for low frequencies, it is stable (it does not tend to infinity, as opposed to the trapezoidal rule response).

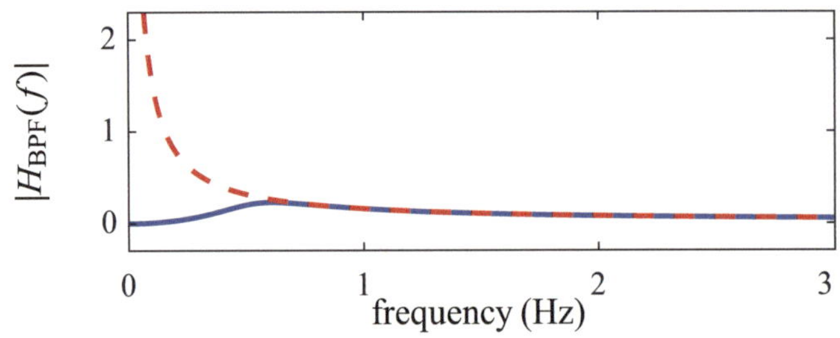

Figure 3. Frequency response of the band-pass filter (solid line) compared to the ideal frequency response of the trapezoidal rule filter (dashed line).

Figure 4 illustrates the process of computing compression depth with this method. First, the acceleration signal $a(t)$ (first panel) is processed with the band-pass filter to obtain velocity, $v(t)$ (second panel). Then, this process is repeated with the velocity to obtain the computed compression depth signal $s_c(t)$ (third panel). Because of the suppression of the low-frequency components and the waveform distortion caused by the filtering process, $s_c(t)$ and the reference compression depth signal $s(t)$ (fourth panel) have different waveforms. However, compression depth and rate can be easily computed by applying a peak detector to $s_c(t)$ and measuring the peak-to-peak amplitude and the distance between the peaks, respectively. Compression rate is computed as the inverse of the distance between two consecutive peaks,

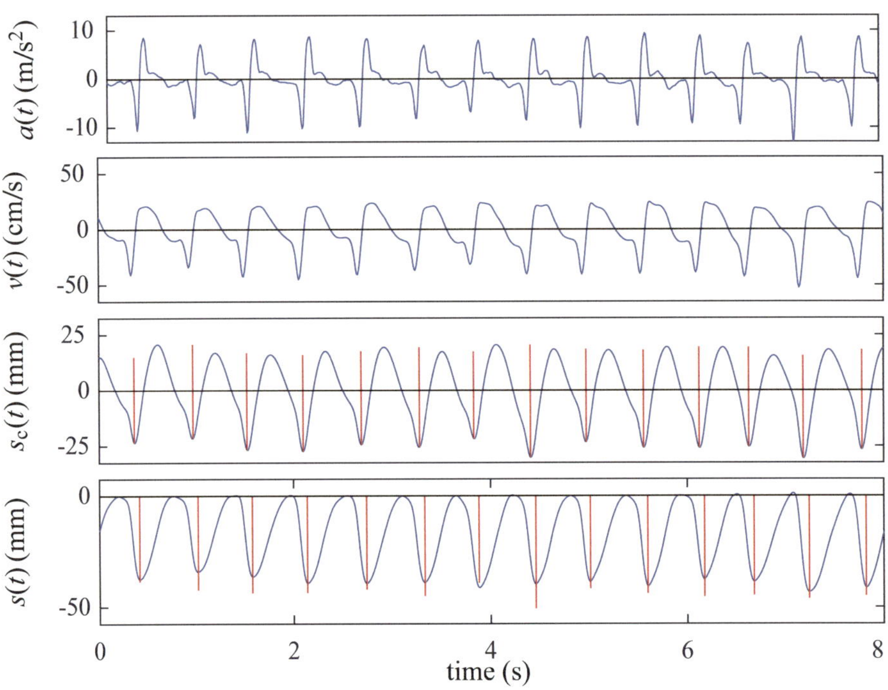

Figure 4. BPF method, based on band-pass filtering.

expressed in compressions per minute (cpm). In **Figure 4**, the detected compressions and their corresponding depths are depicted by vertical lines in the third and fourth panels.

3.2.2. *Detection of zero-crossing instants in the velocity signal (ZCV)*

In this second method, the compression rate and depth values are directly calculated from the velocity signal, without computing the compression depth signal. For that purpose, the band-pass filter described in the previous section is applied to the acceleration once to obtain the velocity signal. The resulting signal is quite stable and can be processed to identify the zero-crossing instants from positive to negative, which represent the onset of each compression cycle (marked by circles in the second panel of **Figure 5**) and the zero-crossing instants from negative to positive, which correspond to the points of maximum displacement of the chest (marked by crosses in the second panel). For each compression cycle, the compression depth is computed as the area of the velocity signal between the onset and the maximum displacement point (shadowed in the second panel of the figure). Finally, the rate of the chest compressions can be computed as the inverse of the interval between two consecutive zero-crossing instants from positive to negative. In the bottom panel of **Figure 5**, the computed depth values (represented by vertical lines) are drawn over the reference compression depth signal for comparison.

3.2.3. *Spectral analysis of the acceleration signal*

In this third method, neither the compression depth nor the velocity signal is computed by integration. Instead of that, average compression rate and depth values are computed every 2 s by applying spectral analysis to the acceleration signal [17]. The basis of this method is the assumption that during short intervals with continuous chest compressions, the acceleration

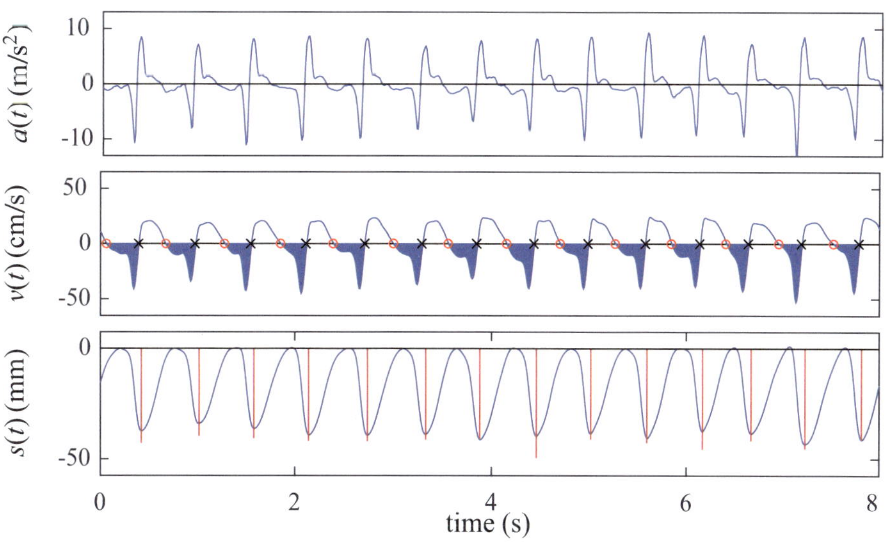

Figure 5. ZCV method, based on the analysis of velocity.

and the displacement signals are quasi-periodic. Consequently, both signals can be modeled as a periodic acceleration and a periodic depth, with a fundamental frequency that represents the average frequency of the chest compressions during the interval. We modeled each 2-s segment of the acceleration and displacement signals using the first three harmonics of their Fourier series representation, without considering the direct current component. **Figure 6** illustrates the procedure followed to apply this method. We first computed the fast Fourier transform (FFT) of the windowed acceleration signal and estimated the module and phase of the three first harmonic components of the acceleration. In the example shown in the figure, the selected window is shaded in the first panel, and its FFT with the identified harmonics is shown in the second panel. Taking into account that acceleration is the second derivative of displacement, when both signals are modeled as periodic, the amplitudes and phases of the spectral components of the compression depth can be derived from the ones of the acceleration. Using these values, a periodic version of the chest displacement during the analysis window can be reconstructed. This last step is represented in the third panel of **Figure 6**. The reference compression depth signal is plotted using a solid line, and the reconstructed signal for the selected window is represented by a dashed line. The reconstructed signal is periodic; i.e., it has the same amplitude for all the compressions, which represent the average compression depth during the analysis window. Average compression rate for each 2-s analysis window is computed from the fundamental frequency of the acceleration, f_{cc}.

3.3. Results

Panel (A) of **Figure 7** shows the boxplots of the error in the estimation of compression depth for each of the methods. On each box, the central mark is the median, and the edges of the box

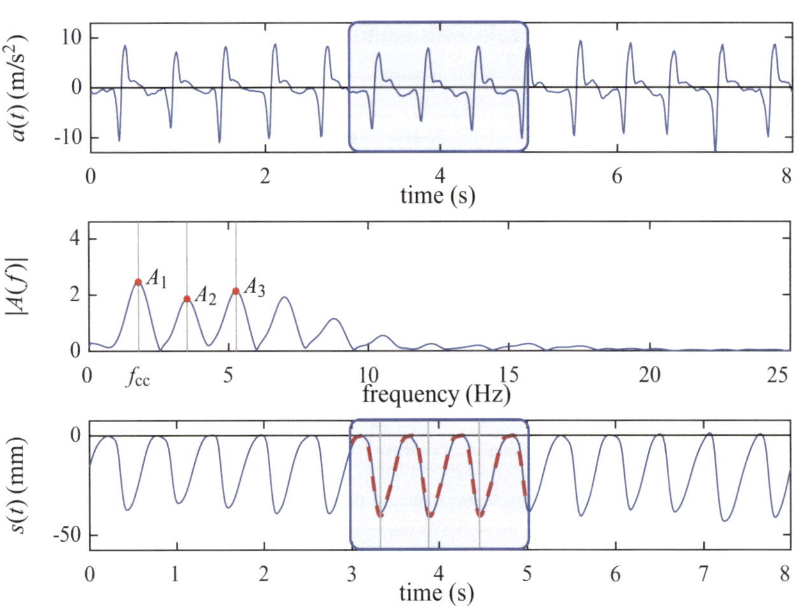

Figure 6. SAA method, based on the spectral analysis of the acceleration.

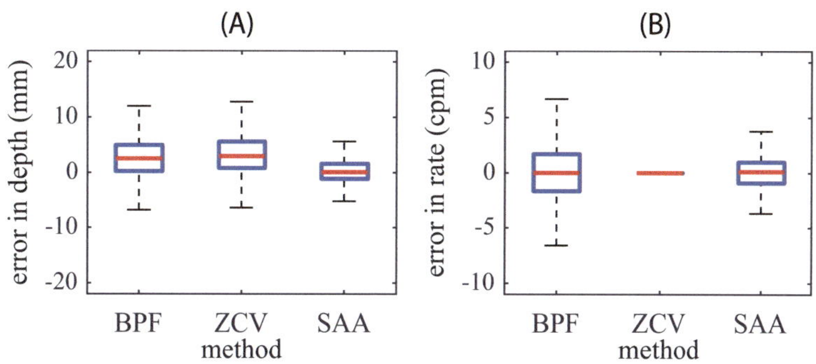

Figure 7. Boxplots of the global error in depth (A) and in rate (B) for the three methods.

are the percentiles 25 and 75, P_{25} and P_{75}, respectively. The whiskers extend to the most extreme data points not considered outliers i.e., within the ±1.5 interquartile range (IQR) interval. Differences in the errors between methods were statistically significant ($p<0.001$). SAA provided the highest accuracy, while BPF and ZCV displayed a slight tendency to overestimate depth values. Median (P_{25}-P_{75}) unsigned percent error in depth calculation for each method was 5.9 (2.8–10.3), 6.3 (2.9–11.3), and 2.5 (1.2–4.4)%.

Boxplots of the error in rate estimation are represented in panel (B) of **Figure 7**. For the ZCV method, errors were clearly concentrated around zero. Median (P_{25}-P_{75}) unsigned percent error in rate calculation was 1.7 (0.0–2.3), 0.0 (0.0–2.0), and 0.9 (0.4–1.6)% for BPF, ZCV, and SAA, respectively. Differences between methods in error in rate estimation were not statistically significant ($p=0.49$).

3.4. Discussion

This section presents three strategies for feedback on the rate and depth of chest compressions during CPR by processing exclusively the acceleration signal and assesses their accuracy in a simulated manikin scenario.

The BPF and ZCV tended to overestimate chest compression depth and presented errors above 5 mm in 25% of the compressions. The SAA method, in contrast, was very accurate and not biased, with an error above 5 mm in only about 5% of the cases.

Percent error in rate estimation was very low for the three methods (median of 1.7, 0.0, and 0.9% for BPF, ZCV, and SAA, respectively). Errors of BPF and ZCV methods were mainly caused by the filter transient, particularly at the beginning of each compression series. This influence was higher for the BPF method, in which the filter was applied twice.

Most current CPR feedback devices rely on accelerometry and double integration to estimate chest compression depth. Manufacturers have designed different solutions for the instability problem, often protected by patent rights, based on either using additional pressure or force sensors to detect the onset of each compression cycle, or on advanced filtering techniques requiring reference signals. All these solutions lead to complex devices, limiting their widespread use in the practice, especially for bystanders and first responders to a cardiac arrest.

The methods discussed in this section are based solely on accelerometry and could lead to simpler, flexible, and cheaper devices. For its simplicity and accuracy, the method based on the spectral analysis of the acceleration might be a good candidate for implementation. To further test this method in challenging scenarios, we conducted three additional studies to evaluate the accuracy of the method: (1) when chest compressions were provided to a patient laying on a soft surface, (2) when the feedback device was attached to the rescuer's back of the hand, or to the wrist, or to the forearm, instead of being placed in the usual position between the chest and the rescuer's hands, and (3) when CPR was performed in a moving vehicle, particularly in a moving long-distance train.

When the patient is lying on a mattress or on any soft surface, accelerometer feedback devices overestimate chest compression depth, [18] as the calculated depth corresponds to the total displacement of the chest, that is, the sternal-spinal displacement plus the mattress displacement. This would lead to erroneous feedback, which could contribute to the delivery of shallow chest compressions. We proposed a solution based on two accelerometers incorporating the spectral method. One is placed on the chest to measure the total displacement of the chest, while the other one is placed at the back of the patient and measures the mattress compression distance. The difference between both measurements will correspond to the actual compression depth. This method presented a high accuracy. Detailed results are presented in reference [19].

Current positioning of CPR feedback devices may cause soft-tissue damage to the patient or to the rescuer, along with wrist discomfort. We analyzed the accuracy of the spectral method when the accelerometer was placed in alternative positions that reduce discomfort: the rescuer's back of the hand, the wrist, and the forearm. We compared these results with those obtained in the traditional position and concluded that positioning the device at the back of the hand was the optimal sensor position. Fixed to the wrist or to the forearm, the sensor was subjected to swinging movements or hands separation from the chest, which caused a large overestimation of compression depth. Readers are encouraged to consult reference [20] for further details.

Finally, we studied the performance of the spectral method when tested in a moving long-distance train. Currently, defibrillators are increasingly being installed in public transportation settings, in an effort to provide an early response to sudden cardiac arrest. Early CPR should be also administered in such scenarios, and the CPR feedback devices could increase CPR quality, but to date how the movement of the vehicles affects accelerometer-based devices has not been sufficiently studied. We tested the spectral method in a long distance train with a manikin setup and compared the results with those obtained in static conditions. Errors in depth estimation tended higher in the train, but no statistical differences were found. Rate estimation was very accurate. Our conclusion was that, as the spectral method does not consider frequency components of the acceleration out of the range of chest compressions (1–10 Hz), movement did not affect performance [21].

In conclusion, the spectral method was accurate to compute chest compression depth and rate in a wide set of conditions and could be used to develop a new CPR feedback device. However, the method is not capable of detecting inadequate rescuer's leaning between compressions. Leaning decreases the blood flow throughout the heart and can decrease venous

http://dx.doi.org/10.5772/intechopen.70742

return and cardiac output. Guidelines recommend minimizing leaning, but human studies show that a majority of rescuers often lean during CPR and do not allow the chest to recoil fully between compressions. This is the current major drawback of any attempt to derive feedback only from accelerometers. For this reason, some commercial accelerometer-based devices use force sensors to provide feedback on this quality parameter.

4. Transthoracic impedance signal for chest compression quality

Most defibrillators, particularly the simplest devices, acquire only the ECG and the TI signal through the defibrillation pads. A straightforward solution for monitoring and providing feedback on the quality of chest compressions could be using the already available signals in current defibrillators. TI measures the resistance of the thorax to current flow. It is calculated by passing an alternate current (usually 2–3 mA at 20–30 kHz) through the tissue, measuring the voltage drop, and calculating the impedance using the Ohm's law. TI is used to check if defibrillation pads are correctly attached to the patient and to adjust the energy of the defibrillation pulse.

Baseline TI is approximately 70–80 Ω in adults, but changes in tissue composition due to redistribution and movement of fluids cause fluctuations on the TI. For example, blood circulation and respiration (or ventilation) generate oscillations of different amplitudes in the TI. In addition, chest compressions during CPR cause a disturbance in the electrode-skin interface, inducing artifacts on the TI. With each compression, the TI fluctuates around the baseline impedance with amplitude varying from 0.15 Ω to several Ohms. **Figure 8** shows a segment of the compression depth and the TI signals recorded during CPR. In the example, two series of 15 compressions were provided, with pauses for two ventilations in between. The oscillations in the TI signal reflect compressions and ventilations. In general, the waveform of the fluctuations induced by chest compressions is very variable between patients and even along each resuscitation episode.

The aim of this section is to explore the feasibility of using TI signal to provide feedback on the rate and depth of chest compressions.

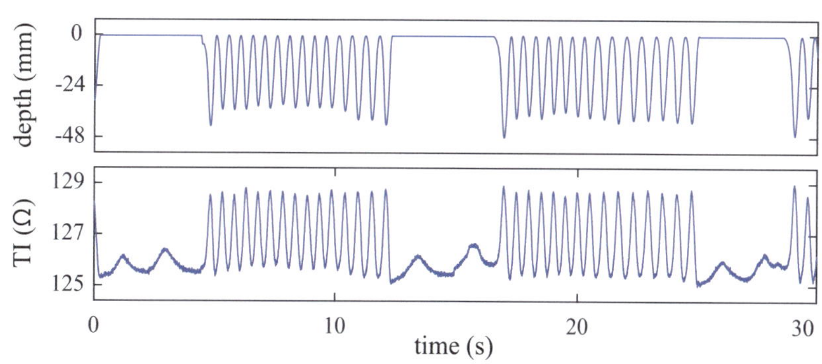

Figure 8. Segment of compression depth and TI signals during CPR. Artifact induced by chest compressions and fluctuation induced by ventilations is clearly visible in the TI signal.

4.1. Use of the TI signal for chest compression quality assessment

Several researchers have investigated the use of TI signal for gathering information on the quality of chest compressions. Some studies focused on detecting the instants of the chest compressions in the TI signals to derive compression rate. Others have studied the relationship between compression depth and the amplitude of the TI fluctuations.

4.1.1. Chest compression rate

The commercial program Codestat (Physio-Control, Redmond, USA) incorporates an automated chest compression and ventilation detector based primarily on the analysis of the TI. The program annotates compression positions and derives the quality parameters compression rate and chest compression fraction (the percentage of time during which chest compressions are provided). Different filtering options allow the user to highlight chest compressions oscillations or ventilation oscillations. Other authors used the TI signal to automatically detect chest compressions in order to estimate the instantaneous compression rate [22]. They found a high correlation between the instantaneous rate computed from the TI and from the compression depth signal. The TI was used also to detect pauses in chest compressions [23] and could be used to measure chest compression fraction.

A comprehensive study that aimed to determine the feasibility of a generic algorithm for feedback on chest compression rate using the TI signal recorded through the defibrillation pads was recently published [24]. Out-of-hospital cardiac arrest episodes were collected equally from three different emergency services and different defibrillator models. The algorithm for computing compression rate was based on the spectral analysis of the TI signal. The gold standard was obtained from reference signals such as the force or the ECG. This approach was accurate under different device front ends and a wide range of conditions, proving the generality of the results. The availability of feedback on the rate of chest compressions could have a significant impact on the quality of CPR, especially in basic life-support emergency systems.

4.1.2. Chest compression depth

Regarding the relationship between chest compression depth and the amplitude of the fluctuations induced in the TI, contradictory results have been found in the literature. An experimental study conducted with swine reported higher amplitudes in the TI oscillations for higher compression depths [25]. Another study using porcine models reported high correlations between TI and systolic blood pressure, end-tidal CO2, cardiac output, and carotid flow [26]. Two clinical studies suggested the potential of TI to identify adequate chest compression depth in patients under cardiac arrest [27, 28]. However, none of those studies included any objective measurement of the actual compression depth; i.e., no gold standard was used to validate the hypothesis. In subsequent studies in which a reference compression depth was included, contradictory results were found, and limited details were provided on the methods and the data analyzed [29, 30]. Finally, a prospective, experimental study with swine by Zhang et al. [31] reported a high correlation between TI and both the compression depth and the coronary perfusion. They found significant differences in the TI fluctuation amplitude between adequate and shallow chest compressions, and a strong linear relationship between TI amplitude and compression depth. Authors concluded that changes in the TI had the potential to

http://dx.doi.org/10.5772/intechopen.70742

serve as an indicator of the quality of chest compressions. Nevertheless, they acknowledged that further research was required to extrapolate these conclusions to humans.

We present a study aimed to go further into this remaining question regarding TI signal and its application to provide feedback on chest compression quality: Is there a relationship between chest compression depth and TI in humans?

4.2. Estimation of chest compression depth from TI signal

The aim of this study was to analyze the relationship between TI fluctuations and compression depth during out-of-hospital cardiac arrest episodes. First, we analyzed the overall correlation between three morphologic features of the TI and the compression depth. Second, we evaluated the influence of the patient by computing this correlation independently for each patient. Third, we studied the influence of the rescuer, by isolating series of chest compressions corresponding to a unique rescuer-patient pair. Finally, we tried to replicate the experiments by Zhang et al., focusing on the correlation analysis with series of optimal and suboptimal chest compressions, and we assessed the discrimination power of the TI signals to distinguish between shallow and nonshallow chest compressions.

4.2.1. Data collection

The data set used in this study was collected by Tualatin Valley Fire & Rescue (TVF&R), a first response advanced life-support fire agency serving 11 incorporated cities in Oregon, USA. It comprised 623 out-of-hospital cardiac arrest episodes recorded during CPR. The compression depth and TI signals were available for 189 of the 623 episodes. We extracted 60 episodes containing both signals concurrently, with a minimum of 1000 chest compressions per episode. Only chest compressions included in series of at least 10 compressions were considered, yielding a total of 11,667,9 chest compressions. Then, we extracted intervals where the single-rescuer-single-patient pattern was guaranteed. Interruptions in compressions longer than 1.5 s were identified as a possible change of rescuer. We gathered 75 series of this type.

4.2.2. Signal processing and extraction of TI features

Compression depth signal was first processed to compute the maximum depth for each chest compression, D_{max}. The instants when D_{max} was achieved were computed using a negative peak detector with a static threshold of 15 mm. The cycle of each chest compression was then identified using these instants both in the compression depth and in the TI signals. This procedure is illustrated in **Figure 9**, where each cycle is delimited with vertical dotted lines. TI signal was band-pass filtered to remove baseline and fluctuations caused by ventilations and high-frequency noise. To characterize TI fluctuations, we defined three TI waveform features computed for each chest compression:

- Peak-to-peak amplitude, Z_{pp_i}: difference between the maximum and the minimum values of the *i*th TI cycle.
- Area, A_i: area of the TI during the *i*th compression cycle.
- Curve length, C_i: length of the curve of the TI signal in the *i*th compression cycle.

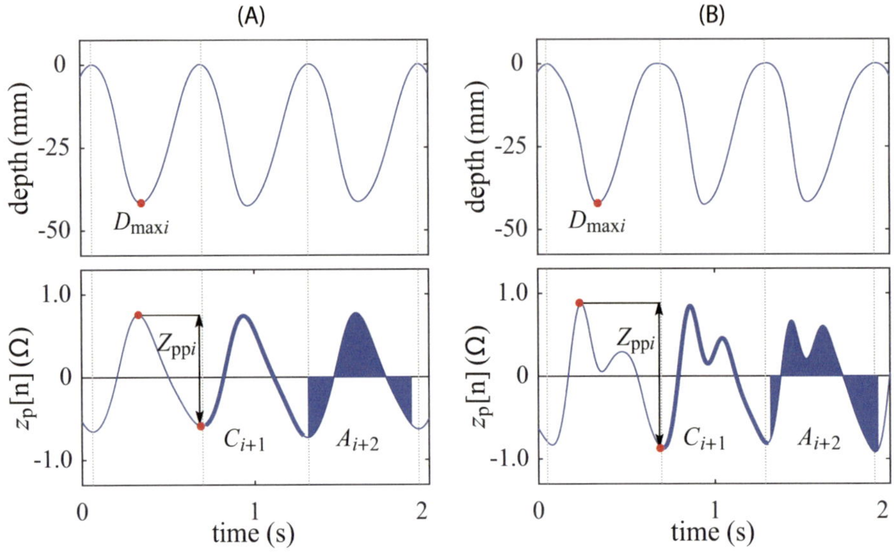

Figure 9. Two examples of the features extracted from the TI signal. The maximum depth is represented in the compression depth signal (top) and the TI features in the TI signal (bottom). Compression cycles are delimited by vertical dotted lines.

Figure 9 illustrates two examples with the extracted features depicted in the compression depth (top) and in the filtered TI signal (bottom). Panel (A) shows quite sinusoidal TI fluctuations, and panel (B) shows a more irregular TI waveform. This is why we computed area and curve length in addition to the peak-to-peak value of TI, as this single feature cannot discriminate between regular and irregular fluctuations. In order to smooth the values of the computed features, the average value of each parameter was computed every 5 s.

4.2.3. Data analysis

The linear relationship between D_{max} and the TI features was tested for the whole population, for each patient independently, and for series of compressions provided by a single rescuer on a single patient. Pearson's correlation coefficient r was computed for each analysis. Univariate linear regression was used to model the relationship between D_{max} and the TI features.

In order to avoid potential variability introduced by the rescuer, we analyzed the relationship between D_{max} and Z_{pp} in a single-rescuer-single-patient pattern. Series with a minimum standard deviation of 7 mm in D_{max} were considered. To avoid bias, a single series per patient was selected, the one with the highest standard deviation. A total of nine series were extracted. Univariate linear regression was used to predict D_{max} using Z_{pp}, and r coefficient was computed for each series and jointly for the whole set.

In order to replicate the procedure by Zhang et al. in their swine model [31], we selected series with optimal and suboptimal series of chest compressions. A series was suboptimal when at least 75% of the compressions were below 38 mm, and optimal when at least 75% of the compressions were above 50 mm. A total of 12 series (one per patient) were selected. They were jointly analyzed computing r and applying univariate linear regression.

Finally, we assessed the discrimination power of the three TI features to classify each 5-s window as shallow (below 38 mm) or nonshallow (above 43 mm) according to the criteria stated by 2005 resuscitation guidelines (valid at the time episodes were collected). We applied a multivariate logistic regression model for the classifier. We split the 60 episodes into a training (40) and a test set (20). The power of the classifier was evaluated in terms of the area under the curve (AUC), and of the sensitivity and specificity in the diagnosis of shallow chest compressions.

4.2.4. Results

Figure 10 shows the scatterplots of D_{max} against each of the TI features for the whole population and the model fitted in each case. In all cases, there was a high dispersion around the regression line. The value of r was 0.34, 0.36, and 0.37 for Z_{pp}, A, and C, respectively. However,

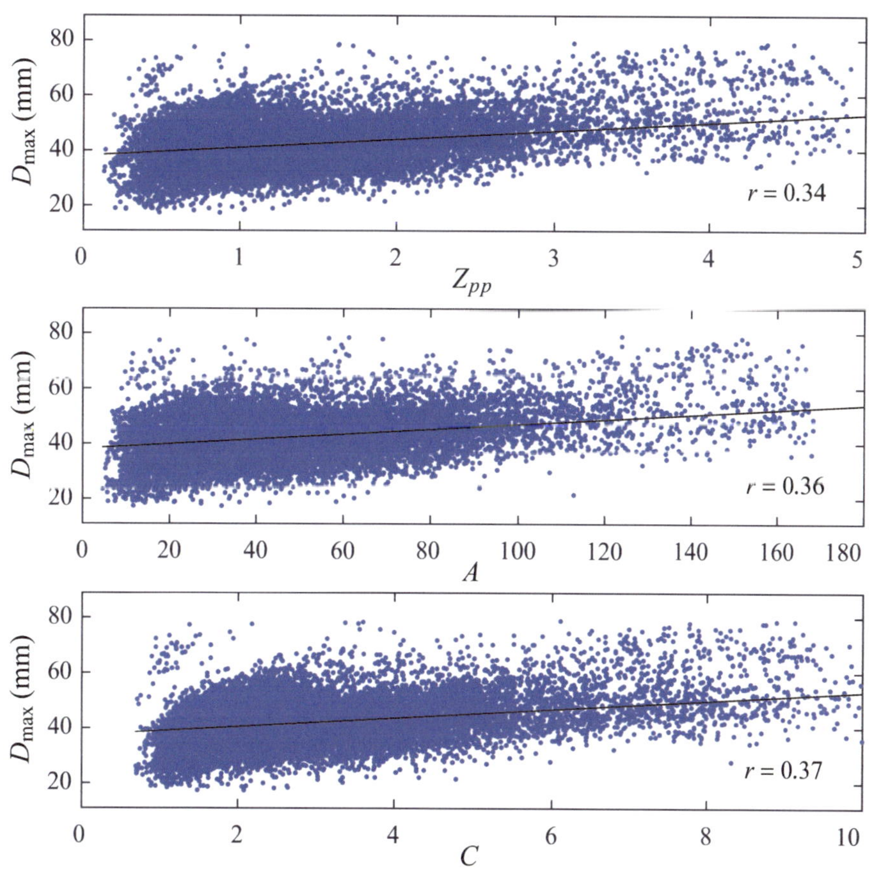

Figure 10. Scatterplots of D_{max} with respect to TI features for the whole population. For each scatterplot, the fitted regression line and the value of r are depicted.

the analysis within patients yielded a median (IQR) correlation coefficient r of 0.40 (0.24–0.66) for Z_{pp}, 0.43 (0.26–0.66) for A, and 0.47 (0.25–0.68) for C.

For the nine series in which the single-patient-single-rescuer pattern was maintained, the individual analysis of each series yielded a median r of 0.81 (0.51–0.83). However, when all of them were considered jointly, r decreased to 0.47.

In the analysis parallel to the one conducted by Zhang et al., we considered the set of twelve optimal and suboptimal series. For the optimal group, D_{max} was 57 (54–63) mm and Z_{pp} was 3.0 (2.5–3.7) Ω. For the suboptimal group, D_{max} was 32 (30–34) mm, and Z_{pp} was 0.9 (0.6–1.5) Ω. We obtained a correlation coefficient of 0.87, quite similar to the 0.89 reported by Zhang et al.

Finally, when analyzing the power of each feature to classify 5-s windows as shallow or nonshallow, we found significant differences between groups, but a high overlap between distributions. The logistic regression classifier showed sensitivity, specificity, and AUC of 89%, 49%, and 0.8 for the test set.

4.2.5. Discussion

Our study included a set of out-of-hospital cardiac arrest episodes with a wide variety of patients and rescuers. The results obtained from the analysis of 14,424 values for each feature showed very low correlation with D_{max} ($r < 0.38$ in any case). Prediction of chest compression depth with any of the TI features was highly unreliable. For instance, for any given Z_{pp} value, the probability of error in the prediction of D_{max} is high because of the wide range of corresponding D_{max} values.

The variability of the results between patients was also high. Sex, chest size, body mass, and pads position have been reported to affect TI baseline, and TI fluctuations during ventilations are correlated with the thoracic fat and thoracic circumference. Our results showed also a great dispersion with respect to the regression line between D_{max} and Z_{pp} from one patient to another. Although, for some patients, little dispersion and high correlation values could be observed along the episode, different tendencies were also found within each episode, showing the influence of different rescuers. In these cases, a single regression model will hardly fit all the values.

With a single rescuer, the dispersion of each series decreased, and linearity between D_{max} and Z_{pp} increased notably. Nevertheless, interpatient factors such as chest/electrodes characteristics of the nine patients caused a low correlation when all the series were considered jointly. This emphasizes the inability to define a confident global linear fit.

Finally, we could replicate the high linearity observed between depth and TI amplitude reported by Zhang et al. in the animal model. We also found significant differences between the optimal and the suboptimal groups, but we also found that for a given value of Z_{pp}, D_{max} varied widely. For a proper interpretation of the apparent observed linearity, we should consider the limitations of the analysis. On the one hand, considering only optimal and suboptimal chest compressions shows a biased picture of human out-of-hospital CPR. When the complete range of compression depths is considered, the correlation coefficient drops to 0.34. On the other hand, the set of patients and rescuers was small (12 patients/12 rescuers in our study, 14 animals/2 rescuers in the study by Zhang et al.). When we included a greater variability (60 patients and 2 to 6 rescuers), higher dispersion was observed and correlation coefficient decreased substantially.

In summary, TI signal can be a feasible indicator for CPR quality parameters such as chest compression rate, chest compression fraction or chest compression pauses. Unfortunately, in this study, we proved that TI is unreliable to predict the key quality parameter of chest compression depth. Nevertheless, we further analyzed, from a practical perspective, the power to discriminate shallow from nonshallow chest compressions, in an effort to achieve a quality feedback method. We tried to discriminate chest compressions <38 mm from those >43 mm. Each TI feature showed different distributions between the two categories, but high overlap between them. The results of the logistic regression classifier allowed us to conclude that it is not possible to safely identify shallow chest compressions using the TI signal.

5. Conclusions

During CPR, the quality of chest compressions is related to patient's survival. Feedback devices guide the rescuers toward target compression depth and rate, and contribute to increase the CPR quality. This chapter explored new alternatives to provide feedback on the quality of chest compressions during CPR. Two strategies were studied: the use of the chest acceleration, which can be acquired using an extra pad placed on the chest of the patient during CPR and the use of the transthoracic impedance (TI) signal, which is acquired by current defibrillators through defibrillation pads. Chest acceleration can be used to accurately compute chest compression rate and depth in a wide range of conditions. TI, in contrast, can be used to accurately compute chest compression rate, but not to identify too shallow chest compressions. The development of simpler feedback devices could contribute to their widespread use and to increase the CPR quality.

Acknowledgements

This book chapter derives from the thesis work *Feedback systems for the quality of chest compressions during cardiopulmonary resuscitation* carried out by author Digna M. González-Otero, under the supervision of co-authors Jesus Ruiz and Sofía Ruiz de Gauna. Several parts of this work have been published in indexed journals or presented at international conferences.

This research received financial support from the Spanish Government through the project TEC2012-31144 and from the Basque Government through the grant no. BFI-2011-166 and through the project IT1087-16.

Authors thank all volunteers participating in the manikin study and the TVF&R emergency medical services providers for collecting the out-of-hospital cardiac arrest data.

Author details

Digna M. González-Otero*, Sofía Ruiz de Gauna, Jesus M. Ruiz, José Julio Gutiérrez, Purificación Saiz and Mikel Leturiondo

*Address all correspondence to: dignamaria.gonzalez@ehu.eus

University of the Basque Country (UPV/EHU), Bilbao, Spain

References

[1] Perkins GD, Handley AJ, Koster RW, Castrén M, Smyth MA, Olasveengen T, et al. European Resuscitation Council Guidelines for Resuscitation 2015. Resuscitation. 2015; **95**:81-99

[2] Idris AH, Guffey D, Aufderheide TP, Brown S, Morrison LJ, Nichols P, et al. Relationship between chest compression rates and outcomes from cardiac arrest. Circulation. 2012;**125**: 3004-3012

[3] Edelson DP, Abella BS, Kramer-Johansen J, Wik L, Myklebust H, Barry AM, et al. Effects of compression depth and pre-shock pauses predict defibrillation failure during cardiac arrest. Resuscitation. 2006;**71**(2):137-145

[4] Kramer-Johansen J, Myklebust H, Wik L, Fellows B, Svensson L, Sørebø H, et al. Quality of out-of-hospital cardiopulmonary resuscitation with real time automated feedback: A prospective interventional study. Resuscitation. 2006;**71**(3):283-292

[5] Gallagher EJ, Lombardi G, Gennis P. Effectiveness of bystander cardiopulmonary resuscitation and survival following out-of-hospital cardiac arrest. JAMA. 1995;**274**(24):1922-1925

[6] Wik L, Kramer-Johansen J, Myklebust H, Sørebø H, Svensson L, Fellows B, et al. Quality of cardiopulmonary resuscitation during out-of-hospital cardiac arrest. JAMA. 2005;**293**(3): 299-304

[7] Koster WK, Baubin MA, Bossaert LL, Caballero A, Cassan P, Castrén M, et al. European Resuscitation Council Guidelines for Resuscitation 2010 Section 2 Adult basic life support and use of automated external. Resuscitation. 2010;**81**(10):1277-1292

[8] Perkins GD, Travers AH, Berg RA, Castren M, Considine J, Escalante R, et al. Part 3: Adult basic life support and automated external defibrillation: 2015 International Consensus on Cardiopulmonary Resuscitation and iovascular Care Science with Treatment Recommendations. Resuscitation. 2015;**95**:e43-e69

[9] Perkins GD, Augré C, Rogers H, Allan M, Thickett DR. CPREzy^{TM}: An evaluation during simulated cardiac arrest on a hospital bed. Resuscitation. 2005;**64**(1):103-108

[10] Abella BS, Edelson DP, Kim S, Retzer E, Myklebust H, Barry AM, et al. CPR quality improvement during in-hospital cardiac arrest using a real-time audiovisual feedback system. Resuscitation. 2007;**73**(1):54-61

[11] Pozner CN, Almozlino A, Elmer J, Poole S, McNamara D, Barash D. Cardiopulmonary resuscitation feedback improves the quality of chest compression provided by hospital health care professionals. The American Journal of Emergency Medicine. 2011;**29**(6):618-625

[12] Yeung J, Meeks R, Edelson D, Gao F, Soar J, Perkins GD. The use of CPR feedback/prompt devices during training and CPR performance: A systematic review. Resuscitation. 2009;**80**(7):743-751

[13] Gruber J, Stumpf D, Zapletal B, Neuhold S, Fischer H. Real-time feedback systems in CPR. Trends in Anaesthesia and Critical Care. 2012;**2**(6):287-294

[14] Gruben KG, Guerci AD, Halperin HR, Popel AS, Tsitlik JE. Sternal force-displacement relationship during cardiopulmonary resuscitation. Journal of Biomechanical Engineering. 1993;**115**(2):195-201

[15] Tomlinson AE, Nysaether J, Kramer-Johansen J, Steen PA, Dorph E. Compression force–depth relationship during out-of-hospital cardiopulmonary resuscitation. Resuscitation. 2007;**72**(3):364-370

[16] Ruiz de Gauna S, González-Otero DM, Ruiz J, Russell JK. Feedback on the rate and depth of chest compressions during cardiopulmonary resuscitation using only accelerometers. PLoS ONE. 2016;**11**(3):e0150139

[17] González Otero DM, Ruiz JM, Ruiz de GS, Irusta U, Ayala U, Alonso E. A new method for feedback on the quality of chest compressions during cardiopulmonary resuscitation. BioMed Research Iinternational. 2014; Article ID 865967

[18] Perkins GD, Kocierz L, Smith SCL, McCulloch RA, Davies RP. Compression feedback devices over estimate chest compression depth when performed on a bed. Resuscitation. 2009;**80**(1):79-82

[19] Ruiz de Gauna S, González-Otero DM, Ruiz J, Gutierrez JJ, Russell JK. A feasibility study for measuring accurate chest compression depth and rate on soft surfaces using two accelerometers and spectral analysis. Biomed Research International. 2016;Article ID 6596040

[20] Ruiz de Gauna S, González-Otero DM, Ruiz J, Chicote B, Ruiz J, Russell JK. Estimation of the chest compression depth using an accelerometer positioned on the rescuer's back of the hand or forearm. Resuscitation. 2015;**96**(S1):16

[21] González-Otero DM, Ruiz de Gauna S, Ruiz JM, Chicote B, Plaza S. Feasibility of compression depth estimation from the acceleration signal during cardiopulmonary resuscitation in long-distance trains. Computing in Cardiology Conference (CinC). 6-9 Sept, 2015;**42**:533-536

[22] Aramendi E, Ayala U, Irusta U, Alonso E, Eftestøl T, Kramer- Johansen J. Suppression of the cardiopulmonary resuscitation artefacts using the instantaneous chest compression rate extracted from the thoracic impedance. Resuscitation. 2012;**83**(6):692-698

[23] González-Otero DM, Ruiz de Gauna S, Ruiz JM, Ayala U, Alonso E. Automatic detection of chest compression pauses using the transthoracic impedance signal. Computing in Cardiology Conference (CinC). 9-12, Sept 2012;**39**:21-24

[24] González-Otero DM, Ruiz de Gauna S, Ruiz J, Daya M, Wik L, Russell JK, et al. Chest compression rate feedback based on transthoracic impedance. Resuscitation. 2015;**93**: 82-88

[25] Brody D, Di Maio R, Crawford P, Navarro C, Anderson J. The impedance cardiogram amplitude as an indicator of cardiopulmonary resuscitation efficacy in a porcine model of cardiac arrest. Journal of the American College of Cardiology. 2011;**57**(14):E1134

[26] Howe AJ, Di Maio R, Crawford P, Brody D, Navarro C, McEneaney D, et al. The impedance cardiogram as an indicator of chest compression efficacy during cardiopulmonary resuscitation in a porcine model: correlation with physiological parameters and comparison with compression depth and thrust. Circulation. 2011;**124**(21 Supplement):A54

[27] Di Maio RC, Navarro C, Cromie N, Anderson J, Adgey A. The impedance cardiogram is an indicator of CPR effectiveness for out-of-hospital cardiac arrest victims. European Heart Journal Supplement. 2010;**12**:F123

[28] Navarro C, Cromie N, Maio RD, Anderson J. Use of the impedance cardiogram in public access defibrillators as an indicator of cardiopulmonary resuscitation effectiveness. Computing in Cardiology (CinC). 18-21, Sept 2011;**8**:601-604

[29] Di Maio R, Howe A, McCanny P, Crispino-O'Connell G, McIntyre A, Patton M, et al. Is the impedance cardiograma potential indicator of effective external cardiac massage in a human model? A study to establish if there is a linear correlation between the impedance cardiogram and depth in a cardiac arrest setting. Circulation. 2012;**126**(21 Supplement): A94

[30] Aramendi E, Ayala U, Irusta U, Alonso E. Use of the transthoracic impedance to determine CPR quality parameters. Resuscitation. 2010;**81**(2):S52

[31] Zhang H, Yang Z, Huang Z, Chen B, Zhang L, Li H, et al. Transthoracic impedance for the monitoring of quality of manual chest compression during cardiopulmonary resuscitation. Resuscitation. 2012;**83**(10):1281-1286

Chapter 7

Focused Sonography in Cardiac Arrest

Marc Delaney, Bjorn Flora and Sahar Ahmad

Additional information is available at the end of the chapter

http://dx.doi.org/10.5772/intechopen.70585

Abstract

Cardiac arrest (CA) is a high mortality event where the ability for clinicians to diagnose etiology and assess for intervention has a direct impact on patient outcomes. Bedside ultrasound (US) has emerged in current literature as a clinical tool to aid clinicians in CA resuscitation, though it remains underutilized. Reversible etiologies that can be efficiently diagnosed with US include tension pneumothorax, hypovolemia, pulmonary embolus with acute cor pulmonale, and cardiac tamponade. Other US findings may provide evidence in regard to prognosis. In this review, we present major applications of US in CA, compare existing protocols, and propose future research needs.

Keywords: cardiac arrest, resuscitation, ultrasonography, echocardiography

1. Introduction

Successful resuscitation in cardiac arrest (CA) requires discrete decision-making regarding circulation, airway, and breathing. It is crucial to identify and treat reversible causes of cardiac arrest during resuscitation in order to make decisions that reverse them and more efficiently achieve return of spontaneous circulation (ROSC) [1]. Bedside ultrasound (US) has emerged as an invaluable tool in the diagnosis and management of critically ill patients, including CA [2, 3]. US may aid to diagnose reversible causes of CA, such as pericardial tamponade, tension pneumothorax, or hypovolemia; guide procedures and other management strategies for quality resuscitation; and reveal signs that can serve in clinical context as prognosticators for the ability to achieve ROSC and longer term recovery. In critical care medicine, bedside US has been found to be faster and have greater sensitivity and specificity than conventional imaging, which is unavailable during resuscitation efforts [4].

Bedside US remains underutilized in resuscitation medicine as there is controversy as to how efficiently and reliably it can be implemented by clinicians, especially in a high-stakes and time-sensitive setting such as CA. This review will present literature that evaluates implementation of US in CA resuscitation and demonstrates the potential of US to improve patient outcomes.

2. Intra-arrest: US to identify reversible causes of cardiac arrest

The standard of care for advanced cardiac life support (ACLS) during pulseless electrical activity (PEA) or asystolic CA dictates that providers actively work to diagnose and treat the reversible causes of CA. The following is a summary of the role of US in detecting such reversible causes:

2.1. Tension pneumothorax

Tension pneumothorax (PTX) is a well-known etiology of CA, especially in chest trauma, and can be rapidly reversed with emergent evacuation of air by needle or tube thoracotomy. Approximately 1% of non-traumatic in-hospital CA events are caused by PTX [5]. A meta-analysis showed US to be more sensitive and specific than chest roentgenography (CXR) for detecting PTX, with a sensitivity and specificity of 91 and 98% as compared to 50 and 99% for CXR [6]. Another meta-analysis showed that consultant performed and clinician performed US examinations had similar sensitivity and specificity for PTX [7].

US can also investigate how an identified PTX is altering patient physiology, as clinicians can obtain sub-xiphoid cardiac windows to see inferior vena cava (IVC) engorgement with impaired right heart filling as obstructive physiology. Further research is looking into how the location of a specific lung US finding, called lung point, can be used to quantify PTX size, with initial data showing that lung points found in the mid axillary line of supine patients predicting a greater than 15% lung collapse size as measured by CT with a sensitivity of 83% and specificity of 82% [8]. The convenience and repeatability of bedside US for PTX makes it clinically useful in CA [7, 9].

2.2. Pericardial effusion with cardiac tamponade

Cardiac tamponade is a significant contributor to in-hospital CA, with reported incidence as high as 6% of in-hospital CA [5]. Performing cardiac ultrasound, or echocardiography, during chest compression holds, allows for rapid detection of pericardial effusion. Several studies have validated the diagnostic power of US in this setting, including in the hands of non-cardiologist physicians, with reported sensitivities ranging from 96 to 100% and specificities ranging from 87 to 98% [10, 11]. In the medical literature, outside of the case of CA, use of bedside US to detect tamponade physiology is widely supported. Internal medicine (IM) physicians with handheld US devices identified moderate to large pericardial effusions with moderate agreement (kappa of 0.51) compared to cardiologist-read formal echocardiography [12]. Detecting increased central venous congestion in this setting using the presence of IVC plethora on US has shown a sensitivity of 97% for predicting tamponade, with an understandably small specificity of 40% given the many causes of IVC plethora [13, 14]. Other US predictors of tamponade physiology relate to the enhanced ventricular interdependence seen in tamponade include right atrial collapse (sensitivity of 50–100%, specificity of 33–100%) [15, 16], left atrial collapse (sensitivity of 13%, specificity of 98%), and right ventricular collapse (sensitivity of 48–100%, specificity of 72–100%) [13, 17].

2.3. Pulmonary embolus with acute cor pulmonale

US diagnosis of acute cor pulmonale due to pulmonary embolism (PE) relies on identification of right ventricle (RV) enlargement as an important finding during targeted echocardiography. Outside of the case of CA, other findings of acute cor pulmonale in include septal flattening or leftward bowing and RV systolic dysfunction [18, 19] . The RV:LV end diastolic diameter ratio, D-sign, and McConnel's sign are validated echocardiography patterns of acute cor pulmonale in PE [20]. Of course, these signs are a product of a large flow-obstructing PE altering hemodynamic physiology in the presence of spontaneous circulation, a factor that is not present at CA. However, several case reports and observational studies have reported that, even during CA, PE can still be identified using the same signs of disproportionate RV size and direct embolism visualization in the pulmonary artery, right atrium, or IVC as a homogenously echogenic structure independent of underlying anatomy (suggestive of thrombus presence [21–25]. Such findings may lead to change in management including use of thrombolysis, an intervention that could largely benefit mortality in these patients [26, 27]. Administration of thrombolytic agents during cardiopulmonary resuscitation (CPR) is a controversial and high-risk procedure that can produce serious complications, including fatal hemorrhage, leading to controversy in recommendations and guidelines [27]. Interestingly, studies have added contrast to early case reports of hemorrhage including a recent single-center retrospective analysis of 42 patients that found thrombolysis during CA yielded no significant difference in major and minor bleeding events [28]. In regards to resuscitation, one study on 42 CA patients with PE found higher rates of ROSC in patients who received emergent thrombolysis than those who did not (81% vs. 43%, $p = 0.03$) [29]. While prospective data in this setting is sparse, the largest randomized trial was performed by Böttiger et al. in 2008 with 1050 out-of-hospital CA patients. The trial was terminated early due to futility when no significant differences were detected between tenecteplase and placebo groups in 30-day survival, hospital admission rates, ROSC, 24-hour survival, survival to discharge, or neurologic outcomes [30].

Ultrasound can be used to view the lower extremity vessels for a rapid deep venous thrombosis (DVT) study without interfering with compressions or other resuscitation measures. Studies have shown that bedside US DVT exams performed by clinician-sonographers have similar speed and diagnostic accuracy as compared to a formal US study with a radiologist [31, 32]. One meta-analysis of 15 studies and nearly 7000 patients by Rodrigues et al. in 2016 showed that an abbreviated proximal-focused DVT study, had a pooled sensitivity of 41%, and specificity of 96% for DVT detection compared to 79 and 84% of a relatively time-intensive whole-extremity exam [33]. In this study, the positive likelihood ratio of the limited DVT studies was pooled at 11.9, suggesting a utility of this abbreviated study in settings such as cardiac arrest.

While there is a clear need for further research in this area, many sources are advocating for more widespread use of thrombolysis during CPR in CA patients, especially in those where intra-arrest US helps to diagnose PE early and identify those at the highest risk of mortality [34].

2.4. Hypovolemia

Perhaps one of the most commonly used applications of bedside US is the evaluation of intravascular volume status and prediction of fluid tolerance or responsiveness [11, 35]. During management of CA, imaging of the IVC can help a code-leader rapidly diagnose hypovolemic shock, a tool whose sensitivity and specificity can be enhanced by adding US images of the lung fields and basic cardiac windows in conjunction with US of the IVC [36].

Early studies involved viewing the IVC in dialysis patients and blood donors, showing differences in IVC diameters pre and post infusions with associated changes in vessel caliber with respiratory cycle thoracic pressure changes [37, 38]. The largest meta-analysis in support of IVC US showed a pooled sensitivity of 76% and specificity of 86% for the detection of fluid responsiveness, defined as improved cardiac output (CO) on cardiac catheterization [39]. In both spontaneously breathing and mechanically ventilated patients, IVC US has high sensitivity and specificity for assessing fluid volume and responsiveness, suggesting applicability in the setting of CA, where hypovolemia may be a reversible etiology of arrest [39, 40]. However, US interrogation of fluid responsiveness during CA requires the clinician to be aware of the altered hemodynamic physiology of CA, where there is significant venous congestion and an elevated central venous pressure associated with decreased cardiac output (CO) [41]. In addition, sonographers need to be aware of the comorbidities that decrease IVC imaging sensitivity for hypovolemia, such as an obstructive physiology such as cor pulmonale, cardiac tamponade, or a myocardial infarction with markedly decreased CO [41].

With this hemodynamic physiology of CA in mind, US evaluation of hypovolemia as a cause of CA can still be useful as IVC imaging can be coupled with rapid and sensitive interrogation of the thoracic, abdominal, and pelvic cavities. In these spaces, such a large volume of fluid can accumulate to where this could cause significant hypovolemia if blood loss into these spaces has decreased effective circulating volume [41, 42]. US evaluation for significant intra-abdominal and pelvic fluid accumulation is a widely accepted modality, with sensitivities ranging from 60 to 100% [43–46]. In the setting of CA, this technique can take place without interruption of compressions and has the potential to alter CA management [47].

3. Peri-arrest and post-arrest care: US to guide ACLS

Outside of its use in diagnosing reversible etiologies of CA, US has also been supported by the literature for guidance of interventions in the intra and peri-arrest period.

3.1. US to interrogate cardiac rhythm

During CA resuscitation, one can directly visualize the heart both during compressions and at pulse checks. This has allowed clinicians more insight into the physiology of each patient in addition to data provided by pulse palpation and electrical monitors. US has bolstered the clinical utility of categorizing electromechanical dissociation (EMD) into "true-EMD" vs. "pseudo-EMD." Pseudo-EMD is defined as the sonographic evidence of intrinsic and coordinated myocardial and valvular movement in the absence of a palpable pulse [11, 48, 49]. Several authors have noted that this observation of pseudo-EMD is associated with a better prognosis for ROSC as compared to true-EMD, which shows no contractile movement of the heart. One such prospective observational study involving 49 intensive care unit (ICU) CA events showed pseudo-EMD to occur on US in 55% of PEA patients [48]. This study showed the rates of ROSC were 70% for those in pseudo-EMD compared to 20% for those in true EMD [48, 50]. This US distinction could aid clinicians in their prognostication and decisions to continue or halt resuscitative efforts, with implications to resource utilization. Alternatively, the finding of pseudo-EMD may support a clinical strategy of using vasopressors/inotropes to support this coordinated cardiac activity and better optimize cerebral and coronary perfusion pressures for achieving ROSC. While there is currently no data to support this practice in CA resuscitation, this approach has been utilized with success in shock patients [51, 52].

Similarly, authors have described resuscitative events where "pseudo-asystole" is identified as asystole on electrical cardiac monitor with asynchronous fibrillatory activity of the ventricles on echo, suggesting ventricular fibrillation (VF). In the existing case reports describing this finding, this immediately changed ACLS algorithm as unsynchronized defibrillation was indicated [53–55].

3.2. US to guide chest compressions

US has been suggested as a means to optimize the effectiveness of chest compressions and to increase accuracy and efficiency of pulse check intervals [56]. While there remains a paucity of data to support these uses, the potential demonstrated by early case reports warrants discussion. Effective chest compressions allow for adequate coronary and cerebral perfusion pressure during CA [57]. While ACLS guidelines state the optimal site of compressions is on the lower half of the sternum along the nipple line, some studies suggest significant anatomical variation among structures at this site [58]. One study of 30 out-of-hospital CA patients tested this site compared to three caudal alternatives and found that maximal end-tidal carbon dioxide was achieved at the AHA recommended site in only 1/3rd of their sample [59]. Another study using transesophageal echocardiography (TEE) observed 34 non-traumatic CA patients and identified the anatomic area of maximal compression (AMC) to be over the aorta or left ventricular outflow tract in all cases with a statistically significant linear association between LV stroke volume and AMC distance from the aortic valve [60]. In a swine model of cardiac arrest, animals randomized to have compressions centered over their LV, as identified by transesophageal echocardiography (TEE), had a greater proportion of ROSC and survival to 60 minutes compared to those that had compressions centered over their aortic root [61].

While more research in this area is needed, it is reasonable to predict a role for bedside ultrasound and echocardiography to be identifying appropriate positioning for chest compression efforts, either by trans-thoracic echocardiography (TTE) and/or TEE by viewing the anatomic landmarks directly.

3.3. US to guide pulse checks

Current ACLS guidelines state that pulse-checks during CA resuscitation should last no longer than 10 seconds. Some authors have called the accuracy of pulse palpation into question [62]. One study involving pulse palpation during cardiac bypass surgery (spontaneous vs. non-pulsatile blood flow) showed that, while health care providers with advanced levels of training had decreased decision delay, only 16.5% of the participants (34 of 206) were able to reach a confident decision about their patients' pulse status within 10 seconds [63]. A similar earlier study in basic life support-trained personnel found that although sensitivity of all participants for central pulselessness approached 90%, specificity was only 55% [64]. While these studies have their limitations, they call attention to a potential role for ancillary devices to augment the accuracy of pulse palpation. Case reports have shown handheld Doppler US devices can allow for faster pulse checks in patients during in-hospital CA [62]. Other authors have already reported the utility of US performed concomitantly with pulse palpation to be effective in identifying perfusing heart rhythms [21]. While US in this exact context is not yet well studied, it seems of little risk but some benefit to use US to eliminate some of this intrinsic inaccuracy in pulse palpation during CA resuscitation.

3.4. US for endotracheal tube (ETT) placement confirmation

Verification of endotracheal intubation during ACLS can be accomplished with US of the neck. The usual methods of ETT placement verification have limitations when applied during cardiac arrest. Direct visualization is often not reliable especially if the intubation takes place during chest compressions due to the movements of the patient. Colorimetry methods can be misleading in the setting of a previously insufflated stomach, which is the case with the bag valve mask technique ongoing prior to intubation attempts or prior esophageal intubation with insufflation. Continuous waveform capnography remains as a reliable confirmatory method if this equipment is readily available. It can require time to set up and to evaluate the waveform over several breaths, which can be considered a limitation. US can distinguish an intubated trachea from and an intubated esophagus as each has distinct sonographic findings that can be rapidly attained.

Cadaver studies have shown that neck US findings of "double lumen sign" and "tube sliding" artifact can predict endotracheal or esophageal intubation with 100% sensitivity and 100% specificity [65]. The largest meta-analysis of studies with both adult patient and cadaveric models determined that bedside physicians and house staff had a pooled sensitivity and specificity of 93 and 97% [66]. US for ETT placement is especially useful when waveform capnography is not readily available [67] or if a conventional method is misleading, such as colorimetry-verified placement with continued hypoxia. Several authors have shown that US is quicker than conventional methodologies of ETT placement confirmation, demonstrating an average time to confirmation of 5.8 seconds, significantly faster than capnography at 11.8 seconds [68]. We advocate for enhancing testing characteristics by combining visualization of neck airway structures with lung field pleural sliding and respiratory diaphragmatic motion, which can be performed during pulse check.

3.5. US to guide post-ROSC hemodynamic management

Post-ROSC management includes the immediate initiation of hemodynamic support measures such as fluids, vasopressors, and inotropes. The ability to quickly utilize bedside US to evaluate fluid responsiveness and overall cardiac function can be clinically useful to guide this hemodynamic support.

Goal-directed echocardiography (GDE) is a concept that uses high-fidelity qualitative analysis, without Doppler technology or valvular measurements, to assess targeted cardiac windows in real-time with high sensitivity of identifying marked abnormalities and gross pathophysiology. GDE emphasizes grading LV function as normal, decreased, or very decreased, allowing bedside clinicians to make real-time evaluations upon which to guide management of CA [69]. Current literature supports agreement of GDE interpretations between formal consultant cardiologists and clinician-sonographers at the bedside. One such study demonstrated that, after a brief training course, novice sonographers with hand-held US at the bedside demonstrated 75% agreement with cardiologist in their formal-US study interpretations of LV dysfunction, compared to 83% intra-cardiologist agreement [12]. Thereby, in a CA resuscitation event, when a cardiologist is not always available, a relatively novice-level sonographer is sufficient for diagnostic capability.

Using this concept of GDE, clinician-sonographers can use US to better inform their post-ROSC hemodynamic management including the use of inotropes, pressors, and/or fluid support with the treating clinician acquiring selected TTE views to characterize pre-load and cardiac contractility in the immediately post-arrest period.

4. US for prognostication in CA

An important emerging area of current study in CA US involves using US data in prognostication for survival and neurological outcomes in CA. Despite best efforts during resuscitation, there is continued poor survivorship. The ability to prognosticate the patient's likelihood of achieving ROSC can improve the practitioner's ability to allocate resources and manage expectations of the treating team and patient's caretakers.

The strongest literature supporting prognostic value of US in CA relates to the presence or absence of coordinated cardiac activity as noted by US [11, 48, 70]. Pooled data from over 500 patients showed that the presence of any cardiac kinetics by intra-arrest US had a positive likelihood ratio of 4.26 and negative likelihood ratio of 0.18 to predict ROSC [71]. Another observational study observed the survivorship of nearly 800 non-traumatic CA patients who received US examination as part of their resuscitative efforts upon presentation to the emergency room and showed presence of any cardiac activity on US was associated with ROSC, survival to admission, and survival to discharge [72].

Further areas of research into US in CA prognostication are looking outside the heart, including measuring optic nerve sheath diameter (ONSD) to predict a positive neurological outcome. ONSD was measured in CA patients 12–72 hours after ROSC and at 28 days after ROSC or discharge from the hospital before 28 days [73]. ONSD of less than or equal to 5.4 mm predicted a favorable neuro-functional prognosis as measures by Glasgow Outcomes Scale with a sensitivity of 83%, specificity of 73%, positive likelihood ratio of 3.1 and negative likelihood ratio of 0.23 [73].

5. Bedside CA US is feasible to be implemented today

The viability of using US during a cardiac arrest depends on the premise that non-radiologist and non- cardiologist physicians can obtain and rapidly interpret imaging data about patient anatomy and physiology with high diagnostic accuracy. Among the significant barriers to its implementation and widespread use are lack of confidence in usage of new technologies and inertia against supplementing traditional methods with new tools for guiding CA management.

In response to the issue of implementation, there is much known about the learning curve for non-radiologist and non-cardiologist practitioners to operate, interpret, and apply this bedside imaging technology. Authors from many different fields including emergency medicine, IM, and anesthesiology have conducted research to address this question of feasibility [74]. Multiple studies have shown that, after short-term (hours-days) educational sessions, novice and expert sonographers can perform without significant differences in sensitivity or specificity in challenging US applications such as ventricular function, volume status or cardiac tamponade [75].

Even at the trainee level, it has been shown that US is a technology which physicians can consistently learn. The Accreditation Council of Graduate Medical Education (ACGME) now requires that critical care ultrasonography be a mandatory component of critical care medicine fellowship training, surgical critical care fellowship training, and emergency medicine residencies [75, 76]. It is well established that this can be done successfully with a mixture of didactics, simulation, and hands on training [75]. In a 3 day critical care US course, 300 novice physicians were shown to proficiently acquire and interpret content from thoracic, vascular, and abdominal ultrasonography [77].

Integrating US techniques into CA management is simply a matter of targeted educational sessions focused on image acquisition, interpretation, and immediate application. After a 1-day training course in CA echocardiography given to novice clinicians of all training levels, the rate of US usage in CA management increased from 4.3 to 19.8% and that echocardiography during the CA event altered management in 70% of cases [78]. Another study found that novice sonographers as a part of an ACLS response team were able to integrate US into their management of cardiac arrest with images obtained and interpreted within an average of 8 min from CA alert activation and demonstrated strong image interpretation agreement with expert sonographers upon retrospective repeat interpretation [42]. In an analysis of CA events in the ICU where US was used in the setting of PEA or asystole, images of adequate quality were obtained during compressions in 100% of there were changes in management and diagnosis due to US findings in 51% of cases [48]. These data together suggest that US has significant potential to aid in CA resuscitation management and potentially improve patient mortality, morbidity, and outcomes [42, 72, 79, 80].

6. Overview of selected current CA US protocols

Implementation of US for CA will be most organized if a standardized approach can be systematically integrated into CA management. There are several example US for CA protocols noted to date, including our institutional protocol (**Table 1**). These protocols focus on rapidly identifying causes of PEA/asystole such as cardiac tamponade, PE, PTX, and hypovolemia. Each protocol is designed to minimally interfere with ACLS. Our institutional protocol

Title or author	Views obtained	# views	During CPR, pulse-checks, or both?	Estimated time of protocol	Notes/uniqueness
Ahmad	Lung, cardiac, Abd/IVC, deep venous, tracheal/ ETT	5	Both	Cardiac: 10s Noncardiac: Variable Total: Variable, includes US at pulse checks, compressions, and post-ROSC	Only protocol to include verification of ETT placement.
Niendorff [42]	Cardiac	1	Pulse checks	Cardiac: 10s Noncardiac: N/A Total: 10s	Sonographer ends each exam by voicing "this is a limited screening examination"
C.A.U.S.E. Protocol [41]	Cardiac, lungs	2	Both	Cardiac: <30s Noncardiac: 1 min Total: 1.5 min	Relies on good 4-chamber cardiac views.
P.E.A. Protocol [47]	Lung, cardiac, Abd/IVC, deep veins, bowel, aorta	6	Both	Cardiac: 10s Noncardiac: Variable Total: Variable, US during pulse checks, compressions, and post-ROSC.	The most extensive variety of imaging recommended.
SESAME Protocol [79]	Lung, deep veins, Abd/IVC, cardiac	4	Both	Cardiac: 10–12 s Noncardiac: 40s Total: 50s	Describes addressing most common reversible causes first, includes optimizing depth parameters before imaging.

Abd, abdomen; IVC, inferior vena cava; ETT, endotracheal tube; CPR, cardiopulmonary resuscitation.

Table 1. Comparison of currently proposed organized protocols for cardiac arrest ultrasound.

includes the use of neck tracheal US for confirming placement of the ETT. Most protocols were estimated to take less than 1 min to complete and none endorse interruption of chest compressions beyond the standard time limit of a pulse check. One protocol advocates for saving a video loop of a subcostal view of the heart during a 10 s pulse check, allowing for repeat image analysis [42]. Most protocols emphasize knowledge of diagnostic limitations and careful image interpretation. The complexity of the protocols ranges from 1 view (echocardiography only) to 6 views (**Table 1**).

6.1. Reflections on institutional experience

Our institution is a tertiary care center in New York State, where all inpatient medicine CA resuscitative events are led by senior IM residents, variably with attending. Since early 2014, our institution has incorporated US training into CA management training for these team leaders. In addition, the pulmonary and critical care medicine (PCCM) fellowship program incorporates extensive educational experience in using bedside US in many aspects of critical care, including that for CA. Since the advent of use of this US protocol (**Table 1** and **Figure 1**) for CA, our institution has conducted over 280 CA events and we have implemented use of handheld US devices when a trained clinician can participate. So far, we have received positive feedback from residents regarding the incorporation of ultrasound in CA. Finding a reversible cause has so far been rare. The largest impact has been that the use of US at CA allows code leaders to feel more comfortable stopping resuscitation by ruling out reversible etiologies of CA or findings that represent poor prognosis.

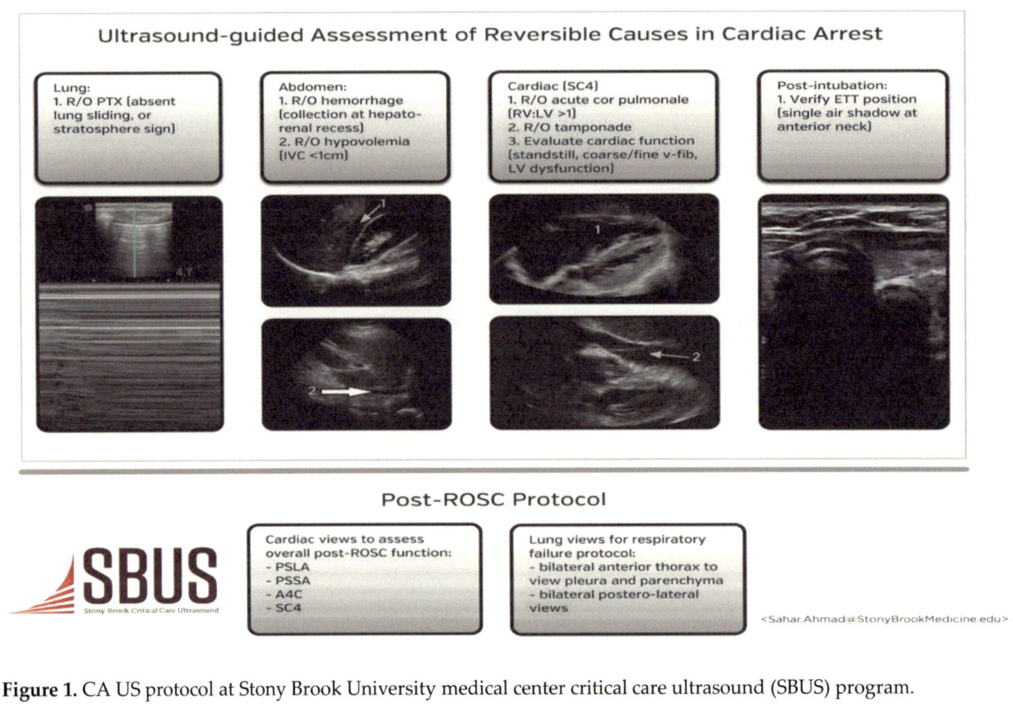

Figure 1. CA US protocol at Stony Brook University medical center critical care ultrasound (SBUS) program.

7. Summary and conclusions

Bedside US has significant implications in the setting of guiding cardiac arrest management. In CA resuscitation, clinicians must make rapid, yet informed decisions about patient care in a fast-paced and high pressure environment. In the case of CA characterized by PEA/asystole, US can quickly assess for reversible causes. US can help physicians better interrogate cardiac rhythm or intrinsic cardiac activity, perform more effective chest compressions, reduce error in pulse checks, more rapidly rule out esophageal intubation, provide more tailored post-ROSC hemodynamic support, and provide assistance in prognostication. CA US allows clinicians to offer a higher level of care quality in concordance with, yet beyond, basic ACLS.

Incorporation of US at all CA may improve cost effectiveness and efficiency of hospital resource distribution. Rapid TTE improved the use of health care resources in patients with CA secondary to trauma, where patients who did not received US had a significantly higher mean cost of care, with an average of approximately $1100 less spent on the US examined group [81]. The prognostic value of US in CA carries an additional resource utilization benefit when considering effects such as ending futile resuscitative efforts earlier and redirecting valuable physician time, hospital personnel resources, as well as medication and equipment costs.

US has become a required part training and accreditation for several medical specialties and it has been consistently shown that physicians can learn US through targeted cumulative educational exposures, even starting at the residency and fellowship levels. It follows that emerging clinicians can be expected to gradually learn to apply these skills to the challenging clinical setting of CA. Most authors advocate for the adoption of a protocolized approach to US in CA as such an approach allows physicians to implement high-yield bedside US in conjunction with ACLS and with minimal interference. Protocolized approaches should include views of the heart to assess cardiac function and for pericardial fluid, IVC for volume status, lung fields to rule out PTX and fluid dependent spaces in the abdomen and pelvis for hemorrhage. Additionally, DVT study and airway confirmation by US may be employed.

Several authors agree that there is a paucity of research to evaluate differences in patient outcomes from US use in CA, therefore true benefits are difficult to assess [82]. Recent survey data identified that there is an existing perception that training in hemodynamic relevant US imaging takes too long, and that only specialized individuals can perform these examinations [83]. However, the literature reviewed here advocate against this criticism. Several authors have shown that time constraints do not prohibit a limited US study and that bedside clinicians can demonstrate success in learning US applications after simple educational interventions. Another barrier is the perception that US devices and sonographers will not be able to join an already crowded space. At our institution, we have found that an US provider, with either a portable or handheld US unit, can easily navigate a resuscitation event without interrupting ACLS. A dedicated sonographer is easily able to adopt to the needs of the resuscitation, change positions and deliver diagnostics to code leaders without interfering with team communications, medication administration, or procedural interventions.

We strongly support the role of US in guiding CA resuscitation management. In light of our and others' experiences reporting US changes management in a majority of CA cases and we suggest that there needs to be support of ongoing research to investigate correlations of US to patient outcomes. US should be part of the standard of care in cardiac resuscitation events as it is currently one of the only means of real time diagnosis of several reversible causes of CA [84].

Author details

Marc Delaney, Bjorn Flora and Sahar Ahmad*

*Address all correspondence to: sahar.ahmad@stonybrookmedicine.edu

Division of Pulmonary and Critical Care Medicine, Stony Brook University Medical Center, Stony Brook, New York, USA

References

[1] AHA MFH, Nolan JP. 2010 international consensus on cardiopulmonary resuscitation and emergency cardiovascular care science with treatment recommendations. Circulation. 2010;**122**:S249

[2] Kendall JL, Hoffenberg SR, Smith RS. History of emergency and critical care ultrasound: The evolution of a new imaging paradigm. Critical Care Medicine. 2007;**35**:S126-S130

[3] Price S, Uddin S, Quinn T. Echocardiography in cardiac arrest. Current Opinion in Critical Care. 2010;**16**:211-215

[4] Lumb P. Critical Care Ultrasound: Expert Consult. Elsevier Health Sciences. Philadelphia, PA. 2014

[5] Wallmuller C, Meron G, Kurkciyan I, Schober A, Stratil P, Sterz F. Causes of in-hospital cardiac arrest and influence on outcome. Resuscitation. 2012;**83**:1206-1211

[6] Alrajhi K, Woo MY, Vaillancourt C. Test characteristics of ultrasonography for the detection of pneumothorax: A systematic review and meta-analysis. CHEST. 2012;**141**:703-708

[7] Alrajab S, Youssef AM, Akkus NI, Caldito G. Pleural ultrasonography versus chest radiography for the diagnosis of pneumothorax: Review of the literature and meta-analysis. Critical Care. 2013;**17**:1

[8] Volpicelli G, Boero E, Sverzellati N, Cardinale L, Busso M, Boccuzzi F, Tullio M, Lamorte A, Stefanone V, Ferrari G. Semi-quantification of pneumothorax volume by lung ultrasound. Intensive Care Medicine. 2014;**40**:1460-1467

[9] Azad A, Al Juma S, Bhatti JA, Dankoff J. Validity of ultrasonography to diagnosing pneumothorax: A critical appraisal of two meta-analyses. CJEM. 2015;**17**:199-201

[10] Lucas BP, Candotti C, Margeta B, Mba B, Kumapley R, Asmar A, Franco-Sadud R, Baru J, Acob C, Borkowsky S. Hand-carried echocardiography by hospitalists: A randomized trial. The American Journal of Medicine. 2011;**124**:766-774

[11] Whitson MR, Mayo PH. Ultrasonography in the emergency department. Critical Care. 2016;**20**:227

[12] Alexander JH, Peterson ED, Chen AY, Harding TM, Adams DB, Kisslo JA. Feasibility of point-of-care echocardiography by internal medicine house staff. American Heart Journal. 2004;**147**:476-481

[13] Guntheroth W. Sensitivity and specificity of echocardiographic evidence of tamponade: Implications for ventricular interdependence and pulsus paradoxus. Pediatric Cardiology. 2007;**28**:358-362

[14] Himelman RB, Kircher B, Rockey DC, Schiller NB. Inferior vena cava plethora with blunted respiratory response: A sensitive echocardiography sign of cardiac tamponade. Journal of the American College of Cardiology. 1988;**12**:1470-1477

[15] Rifkin R, Pandian N, Funai J, Wang SS, Sharma S, Lojeski E, Levine H. Sensitivity of right atrial collapse and right ventricular diastolic collapse in the diagnosis of graded cardiac tamponade. American Journal of Noninvasive Cardiology. 1987;**1**:73-80

[16] Kronzon I, Cohen ML, Winer HE. Diastolic atrial compression: A sensitive echocardiographic sign of cardiac tamponade. Journal of the American College of Cardiology. 1983;**2**:770-775

[17] Ceriani E, Cogliati C. Update on bedside ultrasound diagnosis of pericardial effusion. Internal and Emergency Medicine. 2016;**11**:477-480

[18] Weekes AJ, Oh L, Thacker G, Johnson AK, Runyon M, Rose G, Johnson T, Templin M, Norton HJ. Interobserver and intraobserver agreement on qualitative assessments of right ventricular dysfunction with echocardiography in patients with pulmonary embolism. Journal of Ultrasound in Medicine. 2016;**35**:2113-2120

[19] Poth JM, Beck DR, Bartels K. Ultrasonography for haemodynamic monitoring. Best Practice & Research. Clinical Anaesthesiology. 2014;**28**:337-351

[20] Squizzato A, Rancan E, Dentali F, Bonzini M, Guasti L, Steidl L, Mathis G, Ageno W. Diagnostic accuracy of lung ultrasound for pulmonary embolism: A systematic review and meta-analysis. Journal of Thrombosis and Haemostasis. 2013;**11**:1269-1278

[21] Zengin S, Yavuz E, Al B, Cindoruk Ş, Altunbaş G, Gümüşboğa H, Yıldırım C. Benefits of cardiac sonography performed by a non-expert sonographer in patients with non-traumatic cardiopulmonary arrest. Resuscitation. 2016;**102**:105-109

[22] MacCarthy P, Worrall A, McCarthy G, Davies J. The use of transthoracic echocardiography to guide thrombolytic therapy during cardiac arrest due to massive pulmonary embolism. Emergency Medicine Journal. 2002;**19**:178-179

[23] Volpicelli G, Mussa A, Frascisco MF. Sonographic diagnosis of pulmonary embolism with cardiac arrest without major dilation of the right ventricle or direct sign of lower limb venous thrombosis. Journal of Clinical Ultrasound. 2012;**40**:529-533

[24] Lin T, Chen Y, Lu C, Wang M. Use of transoesophageal echocardiography during cardiac arrest in patients undergoing elective non-cardiac surgery. British Journal of Anaesthesia. 2006;**96**:167-170

[25] Comess KA, DeRook FA, Russell ML, Tognazzi-Evans TA, Beach KW. The incidence of pulmonary embolism in unexplained sudden cardiac arrest with pulseless electrical activity∗. The American Journal of Medicine. 2000;**109**:351-356

[26] Bailén MR, Cuadra JÁR, de Hoyos EA. Thrombolysis during cardiopulmonary resuscitation in fulminant pulmonary embolism: A review. Critical Care Medicine. 2001; **29**:2211-2219

[27] Padosch S, Motsch J, Böttiger B. Thrombolysis during cardiopulmonary resuscitation. Der Anaesthesist. 2002;**51**:516-532

[28] Yousuf T, Brinton T, Ahmed K, Iskander J, Woznicka D, Kramer J, Kopiec A, Chadaga AR, Ortiz K. Tissue plasminogen activator use in cardiac arrest secondary to fulminant pulmonary embolism. Journal of Clinical Medicine Research. 2016;**8**:190

[29] Kürkciyan I, Meron G, Sterz F, Janata K, Domanovits H, Holzer M, Berzlanovich A, Bankl HC, Laggner AN. Pulmonary embolism as cause of cardiac arrest: Presentation and outcome. Archives of Internal Medicine. 2000;**160**:1529-1535

[30] Bottiger BW, Arntz H-R, Chamberlain DA, Bluhmki E, Belmans A, Danays T, Carli PA, Adgey JA, Bode C, Wenzel V. Thrombolysis during resuscitation for out-of-hospital cardiac arrest. The New England Journal of Medicine. 2008;**359**:2651

[31] Pomero F, Dentali F, Borretta V, Bonzini M, Melchio R, Douketis JD, Fenoglio LM. Accuracy of emergency physician–performed ultrasonography in the diagnosis of deep-vein thrombosis. Thrombosis and Haemostasis. 2013;**109**:137-145

[32] Kory PD, Pellecchia CM, Shiloh AL, Mayo PH, DiBello C, Koenig S. Accuracy of ultrasonography performed by critical care physicians for the diagnosis of DVT. CHEST. 2011;**139**:538-542

[33] Da Costa Rodrigues J, Alzuphar S, Combescure C, Le Gal G, Perrier A. Diagnostic characteristics of lower limb venous compression ultrasonography in suspected pulmonary embolism: A meta-analysis. Journal of Thrombosis and Haemostasis. 2016;**14**:1765-1772

[34] Harris T, Meek S. When should we thrombolyse patients with pulmonary embolism? A systematic review of the literature. Emergency Medicine Journal. 2005;**22**:766-771

[35] T Arntfield R, J Millington S. Point of care cardiac ultrasound applications in the emergency department and intensive care unit—A review. Current Cardiology Reviews. 2012;**8**:98-108

[36] Boyd JH, Sirounis D, Maizel J, Slama M. Echocardiography as a guide for fluid management. Critical Care. 2016;**20**:274

[37] Kircher BJ, Himelman RB, Schiller NB. Noninvasive estimation of right atrial pressure from the inspiratory collapse of the inferior vena cava. The American Journal of Cardiology. 1990;**66**:493-496

[38] Cheriex E, Leunissen K, Janssen J, Mooy J, Van Hooff J. Echography of the inferior vena cava is a simple and reliable tool for estimation of 'dry weight' in haemodialysis patients. Nephrology, Dialysis, Transplantation. 1989;**4**:563-568

[39] Zhang Z, Xu X, Ye S, Xu L. Ultrasonographic measurement of the respiratory variation in the inferior vena cava diameter is predictive of fluid responsiveness in critically ill patients: Systematic review and meta-analysis. Ultrasound in Medicine & Biology. 2014;**40**:845-853

[40] Barbier C, Loubieres Y, Schmit C, Hayon J, Ricome J-L, Jardin F, Vieillard-Baron A. Respiratory changes in inferior vena cava diameter are helpful in predicting fluid responsiveness in ventilated septic patients. Intensive Care Medicine. 2004;**30**(9):1740-1746

[41] Hernandez C, Shuler K, Hannan H, Sonyika C, Likourezos A, Marshall J. C.A.U.S.E.: Cardiac arrest ultra-sound exam—A better approach to managing patients in primary non-arrhythmogenic cardiac arrest. Resuscitation. 2008;**76**:198-206

[42] Niendorff DF, Rassias AJ, Palac R, Beach ML, Costa S, Greenberg M. Rapid cardiac ultrasound of inpatients suffering pea arrest performed by nonexpert sonographers. Resuscitation. 2005;**67**:81-87

[43] Dammers D, El Moumni M, Hoogland I, Veeger N, ter Avest E. Should we perform a fast exam in haemodynamically stable patients presenting after blunt abdominal injury: A retrospective cohort study. Scandinavian Journal of Trauma, Resuscitation and Emergency Medicine. 2017;**25**:1

[44] Dolich MO, McKenney MG, Varela JE, Compton RP, McKenney KL, Cohn SM. 2,576 ultrasounds for blunt abdominal trauma. Journal of Trauma and Acute Care Surgery. 2001;**50**:108-112

[45] Tso P, Rodriguez A, Cooper C, Militello P, Mirvis S, Badellino MM, Boulanger BR, Foss FA Jr, Hinson DM, Mighty HE. Sonography in blunt abdominal trauma: A preliminary progress report. Journal of Trauma and Acute Care Surgery. 1992;**33**:39-44

[46] Kumar S, Bansal VK, Muduly DK, Sharma P, Misra MC, Chumber S, Singh S, Bhardwaj D. Accuracy of focused assessment with sonography for trauma (fast) in blunt trauma abdomen—A prospective study. The Indian Journal of Surgery. 2015;**77**:393-397

[47] Testa A, Cibinel G, Portale G, Forte P, Giannuzzi R, Pignataro G, Silveri NG. The proposal of an integrated ultrasonographic approach into the als algorithm for cardiac arrest: The pea protocol. European Review for Medical and Pharmacological Sciences. 2010;**14**:77-88

[48] Flato UAP, Paiva EF, Carballo MT, Buehler AM, Marco R, Timerman A. Echocardiography for prognostication during the resuscitation of intensive care unit patients with non-shockable rhythm cardiac arrest. Resuscitation. 2015;**92**:1-6

[49] Paradis NA, Martin GB, Goetting MG, Rivers EP, Feingold M, Nowak RM. Aortic pressure during human cardiac arrest. Identification of pseudo-electromechanical dissociation. CHEST. 1992;**101**:123-128

[50] Salen P, Melniker L, Chooljian C, Rose JS, Alteveer J, Reed J, Heller M. Does the presence or absence of sonographically identified cardiac activity predict resuscitation outcomes of cardiac arrest patients? The American Journal of Emergency Medicine. 2005;**23**:459-462

[51] Bouferrache K, Amiel J-B, Chimot L, Caille V, Charron C, Vignon P, Vieillard-Baron A. Initial resuscitation guided by the surviving sepsis campaign recommendations and early echocardiographic assessment of hemodynamics in intensive care unit septic patients: A pilot study. Critical Care Medicine. 2012;**40**:2821-2827

[52] Vieillard-Baron A, Prin S, Chergui K, Dubourg O, Jardin F. Hemodynamic instability in sepsis: Bedside assessment by doppler echocardiography. American Journal of Respiratory and Critical Care Medicine. 2003;**168**:1270-1276

[53] Limb C, Siddiqui MA. Apparent asystole: Are we missing a lifesaving opportunity? BMJ Case Reports. 2015;**2015**:bcr2014208364

[54] Amaya SC, Langsam A. Ultrasound detection of ventricular fibrillation disguised as asystole. Annals of Emergency Medicine. 1999;**33**:344-346

[55] Querellou E, Meyran D, Petitjean F, Le Dreff P, Maurin O. Ventricular fibrillation diagnosed with trans-thoracic echocardiography. Resuscitation. 2009;**80**:1211-1213

[56] Ramarapu S. Complete neurological recovery after transesophageal echocardiography-guided diagnosis and management of prolonged cardiopulmonary resuscitation. A&A Case Reports. 2015;**5**:192-194

[57] Georgiou M, Papathanassoglou E, Xanthos T. Systematic review of the mechanisms driving effective blood flow during adult cpr. Resuscitation. 2014;**85**:1586-1593

[58] Shin J, Rhee JE, Kim K. Is the inter-nipple line the correct hand position for effective chest compression in adult cardiopulmonary resuscitation? Resuscitation. 2007;**75**:305-310

[59] Qvigstad E, Kramer-Johansen J, Tømte Ø, Skålhegg T, Sørensen Ø, Sunde K, Olasveengen TM. Clinical pilot study of different hand positions during manual chest compressions monitored with capnography. Resuscitation. 2013;**84**:1203-1207

[60] Hwang SO, Zhao PG, Choi HJ, Park KH, Cha KC, Park SM, Kim SC, Kim H, Lee KH. Compression of the left ventricular outflow tract during cardiopulmonary resuscitation. Academic Emergency Medicine. 2009;**16**:928-933

[61] Anderson KL, Castaneda MG, Boudreau SM, Sharon DJ, Bebarta VS. Left ventricular compressions improve hemodynamics in a swine model of out-of-hospital cardiac arrest. Prehospital Emergency Care. 2016;**2**:272-280

[62] Schonberger RB, Lampert RJ, Mandel EI, Feinleib J, Gong Z, Honiden S. Handheld doppler to improve pulse checks during resuscitation of putative pulseless electrical activity arrest. The Journal of the American Society of Anesthesiologists. 2014;**120**:1042-1045

[63] Dick WF, Eberle B, Wisser G, Schneider T. The carotid pulse check revisited: What if there is no pulse? Critical Care Medicine. 2000;**28**:N183-N185

[64] Eberle B, Dick W, Schneider T, Wisser G, Doetsch S, Tzanova I. Checking the carotid pulse check: Diagnostic accuracy of first responders in patients with and without a pulse. Resuscitation. 1996;**33**:107-116

[65] Gottlieb M, Bailitz JM, Christian E, Russell FM, Ehrman RR, Khishfe B, Kogan A, Ross C. Accuracy of a novel ultrasound technique for confirmation of endotracheal intubation by expert and novice emergency physicians. The Western Journal of Emergency Medicine. 2014;**15**:834

[66] Chou EH, Dickman E, Tsou P-Y, Tessaro M, Tsai Y-M, Ma MH-M, Lee C-C, Marshall J. Ultrasonography for confirmation of endotracheal tube placement: A systematic review and meta-analysis. Resuscitation. 2015;**90**:97-103

[67] Das SK, Choupoo NS, Haldar R, Lahkar A. Transtracheal ultrasound for verification of endotracheal tube placement: A systematic review and meta-analysis. Canadian Journal of Anesthesia/Journal canadien d'anesthésie. 2015;**62**:413-423

[68] Karacabey S, Sanrı E, Gencer EG, Guneysel O. Tracheal ultrasonography and ultrasonographic lung sliding for confirming endotracheal tube placement: Speed and reliability. The American Journal of Emergency Medicine. 2016;**34**:953-956

[69] Walley PE, Walley KR, Goodgame B, Punjabi V, Sirounis D. A practical approach to goal-directed echocardiography in the critical care setting. Critical Care. 2014;**18**:1

[70] Blaivas M, Fox JC. Outcome in cardiac arrest patients found to have cardiac standstill on the bedside emergency department echocardiogram. Academic Emergency Medicine. 2001;**8**:616-621

[71] Blyth L, Atkinson P, Gadd K, Lang E. Bedside focused echocardiography as predictor of survival in cardiac arrest patients: A systematic review. Academic Emergency Medicine. 2012;**19**:1119-1126

[72] Gaspari R, Weekes A, Adhikari S, Noble VE, Nomura JT, Theodoro D, Woo M, Atkinson P, Blehar D, Brown SM. Emergency department point-of-care ultrasound in out-of-hospital and in-ed cardiac arrest. Resuscitation. 2016;**109**:33-39

[73] Ueda T, Ishida E, Kojima Y, Yoshikawa S, Yonemoto H. Sonographic optic nerve sheath diameter: A simple and rapid tool to assess the neurologic prognosis after cardiac arrest. Journal of Neuroimaging. 2015;**25**:927-930

[74] Alsaddique A, Royse AG, Royse CF, Mobeirek A, El Shaer F, AlBackr H, Fouda M, Canty DJ. Repeated monitoring with transthoracic echocardiography and lung ultrasound after cardiac surgery: Feasibility and impact on diagnosis. Journal of Cardiothoracic and Vascular Anesthesia. 2016;**30**:406-412

[75] Vignon P, Dugard A, Abraham J, Belcour D, Gondran G, Pepino F, Marin B, François B, Gastinne H. Focused training for goal-oriented hand-held echocardiography performed by noncardiologist residents in the intensive care unit. Intensive Care Medicine. 2007;**33**:1795-1799

[76] Greenstein YY, Martin TJ, Rolnitzky L, Felner K, Kaufman B. Goal-directed transthoracic echocardiography during advanced cardiac life support: A pilot study using simulation to assess ability. Simulation in Healthcare. 2015;**10**:193-201

[77] Greenstein YY, Littauer R, Narasimhan M, Mayo PH, Koenig SJ. Effectiveness of a critical care ultrasonography course. CHEST. 2017;**151**(1): 34-40

[78] Preston HM, Collins AS, Reed MJ, Connolly J. A description of echocardiography in life support use during cardiac arrest in an emergency department before and after a training programme. European Journal of Emergency Medicine. 2015;**22**:426-429

[79] Lichtenstein DA. How can the use of lung ultrasound in cardiac arrest make ultrasound a holistic discipline. The example of the sesame-protocol. Medical Ultrasonography. 2014;**16**:252

[80] Salen P, O Connor R, Sierzenski P, Passarello B, Pancu D, Melanson S, Arcona S, Reed J, Heller M. Can cardiac sonography and capnography be used independently and in combination to predict resuscitation outcomes? Academic Emergency Medicine. 2001;**8**:610-615

[81] Ferrada P, Wolfe L, Anand RJ, Whelan J, Vanguri P, Malhotra A, Goldberg S, Duane T, Aboutanos M. Use of limited transthoracic echocardiography in patients with traumatic cardiac arrest decreases the rate of nontherapeutic thoracotomy and hospital costs. Journal of Ultrasound in Medicine. 2014;**33**:1829-1832

[82] Royse CF, Canty DJ, Faris J, Haji DL, Veltman M, Royse A. Core Review: Physician-performed ultrasound: The time has come for routine use in acute care medicine. Anesthesia and Analgesia. 2012;**115**:1007-1028

[83] Eisen LA, Leung S, Gallagher AE, Kvetan V. Barriers to ultrasound training in critical care medicine fellowships: A survey of program directors. Critical Care Medicine. 2010;**38**:1978-1983

[84] Breitkreutz R, Price S, Steiger HV, Seeger FH, Ilper H, Ackermann H, Rudolph M, Uddin S, Weigand MA, Müller E. Focused echocardiographic evaluation in life support and peri-resuscitation of emergency patients: A prospective trial. Resuscitation. 2010;**81**:1527-1533

Chapter 8

Extraterrestrial CPR and Its Applications in Terrestrial Medicine

Thais Russomano and Lucas Rehnberg

Additional information is available at the end of the chapter

http://dx.doi.org/10.5772/intechopen.70221

Abstract

Cardiopulmonary resuscitation (CPR) is a well-established part of basic life support (BLS), saving countless lives since its first development in the 1960s. Recently, work has been undertaken to develop methods of basic and advanced life support (ALS) in microgravity and hypogravity. Although the likelihood of a dangerous cardiac event occurring during space mission is rare, the possibility exists. The selection process for space missions nowadays considers individuals at ages and with health standards that would have precluded their selection in the past. The advent of space tourism may even enhance this possibility. This chapter presents a synthesis of the results obtained in studies conducted at the MicroG-PUCRS, Brazil, examining extraterrestrial CPR during ground-based microgravity and hypogravity simulations and during parabolic flights and sustained microgravity. It outlines the extraterrestrial BLS guidelines for both low-orbit and deep-space missions. The former are based on a combination of factors, unique for the environment of space. In a setting like this, increased physiological stress due to gravitational adaptation and the isolated nature of the environmental demands can affect the outcome of resuscitation procedure.

Keywords: extraterrestrial CPR, microgravity, hypogravity, medical emergencies, cardiac arrest, BLS, space tourism, space missions, space medicine, space physiology

1. Introduction

Cardiopulmonary resuscitation (CPR) is a well-established part of basic life support (BLS) and has saved tens of thousands of lives [1] since its development by Peter Safar in the 1960s [2]. Terrestrial BLS guidelines are developed by national organisations, such as the American Heart Association (AHA), the European Resuscitation Council (ERC) and the International Liaison Committee on Resuscitation (ILCOR). The terrestrial method of performing CPR has not changed significantly since it was first implemented, the locked straight-arm method with the rescuer accelerating their chest to generate the force needed to compress the victim's chest. Other aspects of the BLS guidelines often change and evolve as new evidence emerges, one example being the Chain of Survival, which has recently been updated [3]: (1) immediate recognition of cardiac arrest and activation of the emergency response system, (2) early CPR with an emphasis on chest compressions, (3) rapid defibrillation, (4) effective advanced life support and (5) integrated post-cardiac arrest care [4–6].

Changes in gravitational fields, such as those found in the microgravity of space and hypogravity of Mars or the Moon, pose several practical and logistical problems that will impact on the effectiveness of the CPR administered and affect the outcome for any patient who experiences a cardiac arrest in a space mission. In recent years, several studies have been undertaken to develop methods of basic and advanced life support (ALS) in microgravity and hypogravity, using ground-based simulations, parabolic flights or training for medical emergencies in actual space missions.

It is important firstly to understand some of the physics behind space life sciences. The gravitational force of the Earth, which produces an acceleration of approximately 9.81 m/s^2 at mean sea level and is indicated by the symbol 'g' (small letter), has shaped the anatomy and physiology of human beings over millions of years. The concept of human body G vectors uses an axial nomenclature system that has been the basis for studies related to acceleration physiology since its introduction [7]. The three major axes are longitudinal (Z), lateral (Y) and horizontal (X). The direction of acceleration forces along the axes is called (+) or (−), but in general the positive sign is omitted. The inertial forces are opposite to the acceleration forces, as indicated in **Figure 1**. Therefore, when considering the effects of the G force on human physiology, it is important to indicate the axis and the direction of the acceleration force along it. For example, when a volunteer is performing terrestrial CPR manoeuvres, it is said that they are under the influence of 1 Gz.

It is a common misconception that gravity does not exist in space, either aboard space ships or space stations in lower earth orbit (LEO). Typical LEO ranges from between 120 and 360 miles above the Earth, and the gravitational field at this distance is still quite strong, roughly 88% of that felt at the Earth's surface. Therefore, what is often referred to as 'zero gravity' is in fact microgravity, an important difference to note, and the objects or astronauts seen to be 'floating' in space are in reality in a constant state of free fall. This means they are actually falling around the Earth at the same rate as the orbital speed of their spacecraft, which is approximately 17,500 miles/h (28,000 km/h), providing the same effect that would be given by real microgravity [9].

The prefix micro (μ) derives from the original Greek mikros (μικρός), meaning small. A microgravity environment is one that imparts to an object a net acceleration that is extremely small compared with that produced by Earth at its surface, which can be achieved using various methods, including Earth-based drop towers, parabolic aircraft flights and Earth-orbiting laboratories. Exposure to microgravity has been shown to affect every single body system, and the resultant physiological changes can lead to undesirable health consequences [9, 10].

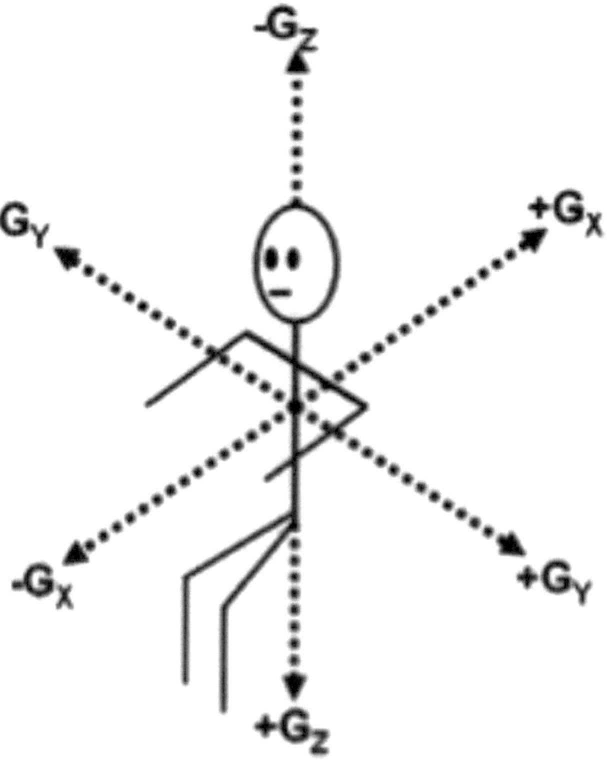

Figure 1. Standard acceleration nomenclature. Note that the arrows indicate the direction of the inertial reaction to an equal and opposite acceleration [7, 8].

The acceleration due to gravity at the surface of a planet varies directly as the mass and inversely as the square of the radius. The Moon is 384,403 km distant from the Earth, and it has a diameter of 3476 km. The acceleration due to gravity is 1.62 m/s^2 (1/6 of the Earth) because the Moon has less mass than the Earth. Mars and Earth have diameters of 6775 km and 12,775 km, respectively. The mass of Mars is 0.107 times that of the Earth. This makes the gravitational acceleration on Mars 3.73 m/s^2, as expressed in Eq. (1):

$$gm = 9.8 \times 0.107 \times (12775/6775)2 = 3.73\text{m/s}^2 \quad (1)$$

Therefore, if a body weighs 200 N on Earth, it is possible to calculate how much it would weigh on Mars. Knowing that the weight of an object is its mass (m) times the acceleration of gravity, we can have W = m × g, 200 = 9.8 × m and m = 20.41 kg. This mass is the same on Mars, so the weight on Mars is W_{Mars} = 3.73 × 20.41 = 76.1 N and m_{Mars} = 7.61 kg.

Some of the physical principles of microgravity and hypogravity have been explained above to clarify some of the common terminology and misconceptions. Throughout this chapter, we will use the terms microgravity and hypogravity. When discussing microgravity, commonly referred to as 'weightlessness' by laypersons, we are referring to being in space either aboard a space craft or aboard a space station and not on the surface of any extraterrestrial body. When talking about hypogravity, this relates to being on the surface of another extraterrestrial body (i.e. Mars, Moon) as these surfaces do have a gravitational field; however, they are weaker than that of Earth's.

This chapter will first present the effects of a space mission on human physiology, considering in particular cardiovascular and pulmonary function and their adaptation to the hostile environment of space. It will then discuss more than a decade of research involving a series of studies examining extraterrestrial CPR during ground-based microgravity and hypogravity simulations and during parabolic flights. It will also outline the essential CPR steps, in the form of extraterrestrial CPR guidelines, to be applied for both low-orbit and deep-space missions, such as a trip to Mars. The rationale behind the creation of specific guidelines for microgravity and hypogravity BLS and CPR is based on a combination of factors that render current traditional methods inappropriate for use in the unique environment of space, a setting in which the human body must adapt to altered gravitational conditions that lead to increased physiological stress, and where the isolated nature of the environment demands greater self-reliance, all of which may hinder a successful outcome when resuscitating a patient.

2. The effects of microgravity on human physiology and its impact on the cardiopulmonary system

Physiological alterations suffered by astronauts during space missions have been observed, reported and studied from the beginning of manned space flight. The microgravity of space appears to affect every single organ and body system of the astronauts, in different intensities and manner, both during short- and long-term missions. The first men to remain in space longer than 24 h were Soviet cosmonauts Titov and Nikolayev in the 1960s. Postflight data collection revealed that the cardiovascular systems of the cosmonauts presented problems in readapting to the gravity of the Earth, with both exhibiting difficulties in maintaining arterial blood pressure levels when standing [9].

During the initial phases of the American space programme, NASA astronauts from the Gemini, Apollo and Skylab missions also showed deleterious signs and symptoms related to exposure to microgravity. Although these early ventures into the space environment were shorter than the missions nowadays, with the longest being a 3-month Skylab flight, it was already evident that the effects of microgravity on the human body would be very challenging. For example, astronauts presented decreases in plasma volume (around 10–20%); red blood cells (space anaemia); bone calcium levels (bone demineralisation); skeletal muscle size and strength (muscle atrophy), especially those that support posture (anti-gravitational muscles and bones); intestinal mobility; immune responses; and sleeping hours [10–13]. Most astronauts also suffered from space motion sickness, which is a common condition, affecting around 70% of astronauts during the first 72 h of a space mission, causing nausea, vomiting, dizziness and light-headedness and consequently decreasing physical and mental performance and overall well-being [14].

Moreover, very early in the manned space flight era, it became clear that the harmful effects on human physiology and anatomy would not be restricted solely to the time spent in microgravity. Important postflight alterations were also apparent after the return of astronauts to Earth's gravity, such as neurovestibular disturbances, orthostatic intolerance and reduced aerobic capacity [15].

2.1. Space cardiovascular physiology

A progressive shift of body fluids and blood from the lower extremities to the upper body occurs in the absence of Earth's gravitational force [16, 17]. Initially, this upward shift increases the central fluid volume, cardiac size (around 20%) and cardiac output. It then leads to a negative fluid balance and reduction of 12–20% in the circulating blood volume [17], which causes a decreased resting stroke volume of 10–20% and a reduced cardiac output with an average of 1.5 L min^{-1} lower than preflight values [18, 19]. These changes are secondary to the reduction in circulating blood volume [20].

This condition has been nicknamed the 'puffy-face and bird-legs syndrome', as the face of the astronaut becomes rounded, redder and more swollen, while the legs become thinner, due to the redistribution of fluids and blood from the lower to upper body. The situation is reversed when the astronaut is once more subject to the gravitational force of the Earth, which distributes the fluid and blood back to its original position [16, 21]. These stages of cardiovascular adaption to microgravity and subsequent readaptation upon return to Earth are represented in **Figure 2**.

Arterial blood pressure and heart rate are more difficult to evaluate during a space mission. While some studies have demonstrated that microgravity can decrease both arterial blood pressure and heart rate [20, 22], others have shown that heart rate, for example, remains unchanged in microgravity [23]. Research is reporting average decrease of 15 bpmin flight resting heart rate and an average decrease of 6 mmHg in mean arterial pressure. These cardiovascular changes were observed when compared with preflight standing values and not supine [22]. In addition, the arterial blood pressure reduction occurred in diastolic values, while systolic blood pressure remained unchanged from that of preflight.

More recently, visual impairment intracranial pressure (VIIP) syndrome has been identified as a health issue occurring in astronauts who have stayed in microgravity for at least 6 months. This syndrome was first reported in 2005, when a refractive change in visual acuity (mainly hyperopia) was detected after a long-term space mission. This finding was further confirmed through evaluations conducted by means of a series of questionnaires applied to astronauts who took part in long space flight missions on the ISS [24]. Very little is known regarding the risk factors and pathophysiological mechanisms involved in space VIIP syndrome. The current consensus within the space flight community is that visual changes and eye alterations (papilloedema, posterior globe flattening, hyperopic shift, choroidal folds) are a consequence of raised intracranial pressures resulting in optic nerve sheath distension. This increase in optic nerve sheath diameter can readily be measured using a simple, non-invasive and low-cost ophthalmic procedure, resulting in an easy way to diagnose this medical condition [25]. However, other factors, such as increased levels of carbon dioxide in the spacecraft, genetic predisposition and ocular and/or brain structural changes secondary to microgravity could also be involved in the aetiology of this syndrome.

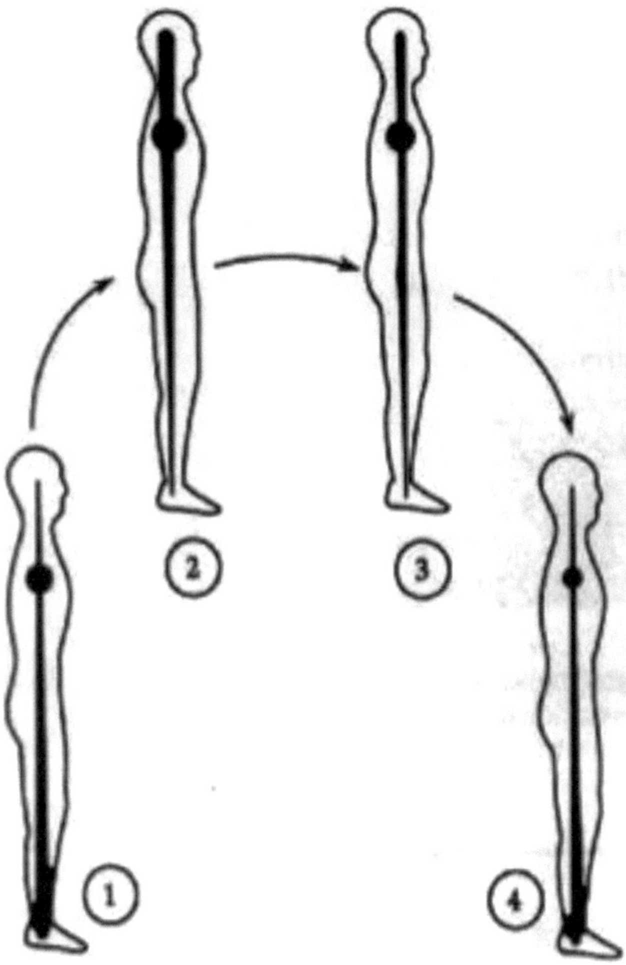

Figure 2. Schematic view of the blood and fluid distribution on Earth (1), after insertion into microgravity (2), during space adaptation (3) and upon return to Earth (4). Note that the puffy-face and bird-legs syndrome occurs in numbers 2 and 3 [16, 21].

Although no serious cardiac events in space have required resuscitation to date, the overall risk of potential cardiac deconditioning developing into a life-threatening illness is approximately 1% per year [26, 27]. Despite this low figure, some documented cases of astronauts presenting disturbances in cardiac rhythm have been observed, such as ventricular tachycardia and prolonged QTc interval after short- and long-duration flights. However, there is little compelling evidence from flight data that space causes cardiac dysfunction or life-threatening dysrhythmias [28, 29]. Ventricular arrhythmias were also reported during the second month aboard the MIR space station [30], and a loss of left ventricular mass was seen during the exposure to microgravity [31]. These factors combined could pose extra stress to the cardiovascular system and, in a worst-case scenario, lead to cardiac arrest [32].

2.2. Space respiratory physiology

Short- and long-term exposure to microgravity produces several effects on lung volumes, capacities and function, which have been assessed during space missions and parabolic flights, as well as in ground-based studies.

Evidence has shown that there is a 4 mm increase in the anteroposterior (AP) dimension of the chest wall at the level of the fifth intercostal space during microgravity exposure. This expansion can be explained by a decrease in weight of the abdominal wall, which allows the sternum to move in a cranial direction. As well as expanding the ribcage, this induces subsequent relaxation of parasternal intercostal muscles, further increasing the AP distance [33]. The effect of microgravity on chest anatomy was also observed during parabolic flights, whereby a displacement of the sternum in the cranial direction was found in microgravity, accompanied by an increase in diameter of the lower rib cage. This change in position of the chest wall was predicted to cause the volume-pressure curve to lie between the standing-upright and the supine-position curves, with the net result of a reduction in lung volumes. In five subjects studied in a KC-135 aircraft during parabolic flight, functional residual capacity decreased by 432 ml during exposure to the acute microgravity phase. Vital capacity also reduced from a mean value of 4.72 L at 1 G to 4.35 L at 0 G. Forced vital capacity and forced expiratory volume in 1 s were also decreased by an average of 2.5% in the 20 s of microgravity per parabola in a parabolic flight [34].

During the 9-day-long Space Life Sciences-1 space mission, forced vital capacity and forced expiratory volume in 1s were significantly reduced on flight day 2 due to the effect of sustained microgravity but were greater than preflight values at day 9. In comparison with standing preflight values, tidal volume was decreased by 15% (110 ml) in microgravity, and this reduction remained during the entire space flight. Functional residual capacity and expiratory reserve volume decreased significantly in-flight by 520 and 370 ml, respectively, when compared with preflight standing values. Residual volume was less during flight by 350 ml, when compared with standing control values. This 20% reduction in the residual volume was unexpected as it is normally fairly resistant to change. It is believed that lung volumes are affected by the changes in intrathoracic blood volume that occurs throughout a mission and by the alterations in respiratory mechanics and cranial displacement of the diaphragm and abdominal content that happens in the absence of gravity [35].

The gravitational gradient affects the distribution of ventilation and perfusion in the upright human lung. This uneven distribution of ventilation and blood flow within the lungs leads to variations in ventilation-perfusion ratios. Cardiogenic oscillations of CO_2 decreased to approximately 60% in amplitude in microgravity [36], and there was also a significant reduction in cardiogenic oscillations of nitrogen (to 44%) and argon (to 24%) in comparison to preflight standing values [37]. Possible causes of the residual inhomogeneity of ventilation include regional differences in lung compliance, airway resistance and the motion of the chest wall and diaphragm. Microgravity was expected to completely abolish apicobasal differences in perfusion, and its persistence is possibly related to other mechanisms not affected by gravity, such as central-peripheral differences in blood flow and interregional differences in conductance.

The diffusion capacity of the lung has been shown to increase by 62% in a parabolic flight study and by 28% in sustained microgravity when values were compared with preflight standing values [36, 38]. The standing-to-supine transition pre- and postflight caused a significant elevation in blood volume in pulmonary capillaries. Diffusing capacity of the membrane was unchanged preflight in the standing-to-supine transition and significantly elevated in-flight in comparison to standing (27%) and supine (21%). In microgravity, the capillary filling is uniform, which is associated with a large increase in the surface area of the blood-gas barrier. Consequently, the membrane-diffusing capacity is substantially raised. This suggests an absence of subclinical interstitial pulmonary oedema in microgravity, as had been previously speculated [38, 39].

The overall effect of acute and sustained exposure to microgravity, although affecting the respiratory system, does not cause any deleterious effects to gas exchange in the lungs. However, there is no current suitable method of accessing arterial blood in space. Consequently, at present, values for blood-gas tensions are usually derived from measurements of respiratory gas partial pressures. To this end, the earlobe arterialised blood technique for collecting blood-gas tensions has been considered for use in space [40]. Access to arterial blood analysis would allow better physiological evaluations and the management of clinical emergencies during space missions, resulting in increased safety for crewmembers.

3. Current cardiopulmonary resuscitation (CPR) practice in microgravity and hypogravity and its simulations on Earth

Although the likelihood of a dangerous cardiac event occurring in a space mission at present is rare, the possibility exists. The selection process for space missions nowadays considers individuals at ages and with health standards that would have precluded their selection in the past. With increased age, less stringent health requirements, longer duration missions and increased physical labour, due to a rise in orbital extravehicular activity, the risk of an acute life-threatening condition occurring in space has become of greater concern. The advent of space tourism may even enhance this possibility, with its popularity set to rise over the coming years as private companies test their new technology. Therefore, space scientists and physicians will have a greater responsibility to ensure space travellers, whether professional astronauts or space tourists, are adequately trained and familiarised with extraterrestrial BLS and CPR methods.

It is currently estimated that the time between the occurrence of cardiac arrest and the performance of ALS on a secured patient during a space mission ranges between 2 and 4 min [41]. However, BLS guidelines highlight that failure of the circulation for 3 min will lead to cerebral damage and that delay, even within this time frame, will lessen the chances of a successful outcome. Therefore, the rate of decline of a patient who has suffered cardiac arrest is dependent, amongst other things, upon the immediate initiation of CPR and the provision and adequacy of such prior to the return of spontaneous circulation, should this be achieved [3].

3.1. Extraterrestrial CPR simulations

The main difference in CPR in hypogravity and microgravity compared to terrestrial CPR is the strength of the gravitational field. In microgravity, patient and rescuer are both essentially weightless. When thinking about the technique of terrestrial CPR, with the rescuer accelerating their chest and upper body to generate a force to compress the patient's chest, it is obvious that this cannot work in microgravity without significant aids. To this end, several microgravity CPR techniques have been developed and tested in parabolic flights [4, 42, 43] and during ground simulations, such as when using a body suspension device system, to test their efficacy [5, 44, 45].

3.1.1. Body suspension device system

Many partial-gravity suspension systems have been designed and used since the Apollo program. The cable suspension method typically uses vertical cables to suspend the major segments of the body and relieve some of the weight exerted by the subject on the ground, thus simulating partial gravity. A body suspension device (BSD) system used to simulate both hypogravity and microgravity was developed by the Aerospace Engineering Laboratory, MicroG Centre, PUCRS, Porto Alegre, Brazil. It consists of carbon steel bars, 0.6 mm × 0.3 mm in thickness, which are shaped into a prism frame. It has a height of 2000 mm, with a base of 3000 mm × 2260 mm [46].

This BSD has been used to simulate microgravity by fully suspending a volunteer and CPR mannequin. A steel cross bar (1205 mm × 27.5 mm) was hung using reinforced steel wiring that gave it the ability to withstand up to 600 kg. A static nylon rope was attached to the steel wiring of the cross bar, with carabineers fastened at each end, which were clipped to the corresponding hip attachments of the body harness worn by the volunteer. A safety carabineer was also attached to the volunteer's back. **Figure 3(A)** and **(B)** illustrates how CPR methods can be studied during microgravity simulations on Earth [5].

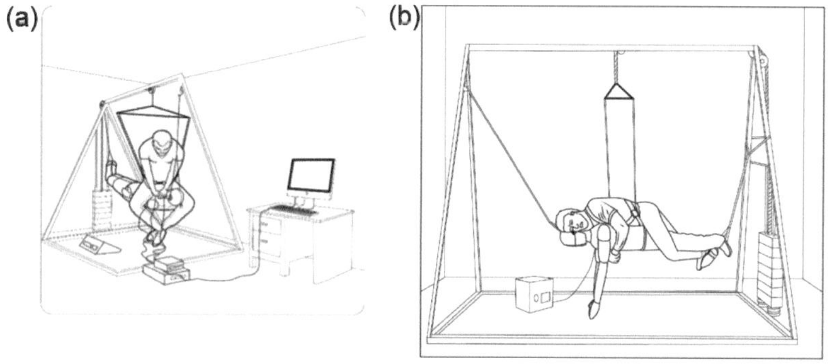

Figure 3. (a) The body suspension device system of the MicroG Centre, with the volunteer perpendicular and the CPR mannequin parallel to the floor, both being fully suspended, simulating microgravity. (b) The body suspension device system of the MicroG Centre, with both the fully suspended volunteer and CPR mannequin parallel to the floor, simulating microgravity.

Another way to simulate microgravity for the performance of CPR is placing the mannequin in the vertical position supported by a wall, which avoids the use of the rescuer body weight during the external chest compressions, as represented in **Figure 4**.

The BSD comprises of a body harness and counterweight system made of 20 bars of 5 kg each. Counterweights were used to simulate hypogravity by partially offsetting the effects of the +1 Gz environment in order to simulate Mars (0.35 Gz) or the Moon (0.16 Gz) gravities. Reinforced steel wire was used in a pulley system that connects the weights at the end of the body suspension device to the volunteer. A carabineer connects the steel wire to the attachment point on the back of the body harness (Fesp P100PGP). The manikin was positioned on the floor during the hypogravity simulation and +1 Gz [6, 46, 47]. **Figure 5** presents a schematic view of CPR being performed during ground-based hypogravity simulation.

The amount of counterweight used to simulate the hypogravity conditions, such as Mars or the Moon, was calculated for each volunteer based on their body weight, as presented in Eqs. (2) and (3) [46].

$$RM = (0.6BM \times SGF)/1G \tag{2}$$

$$CW = 0.6BM - RM \tag{3}$$

Using Eq. (2), the relative mass of a subject in a simulated gravitational field can be calculated, where RM = relative mass (kg), BM = body mass on Earth (kg), SGF = simulated gravitational force (m/s^2) and 1G = 9.81 m/s^2. Eq. (3) gives the counterweight (CW, in kg) necessary to simulate body mass at a preset hypogravity level. The 0.6 refers to the 60% of the weight of the upper body, as the legs are supported on the floor.

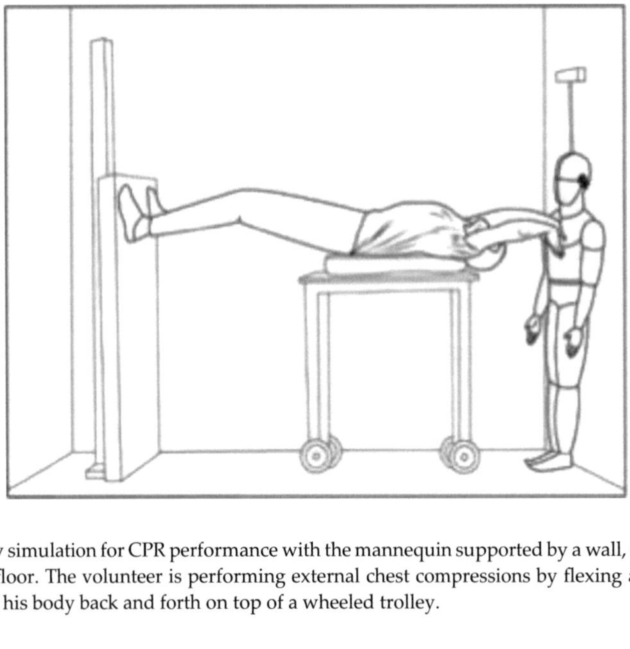

Figure 4. Microgravity simulation for CPR performance with the mannequin supported by a wall, in the vertical position, perpendicular to the floor. The volunteer is performing external chest compressions by flexing and extending his legs and therefore moving his body back and forth on top of a wheeled trolley.

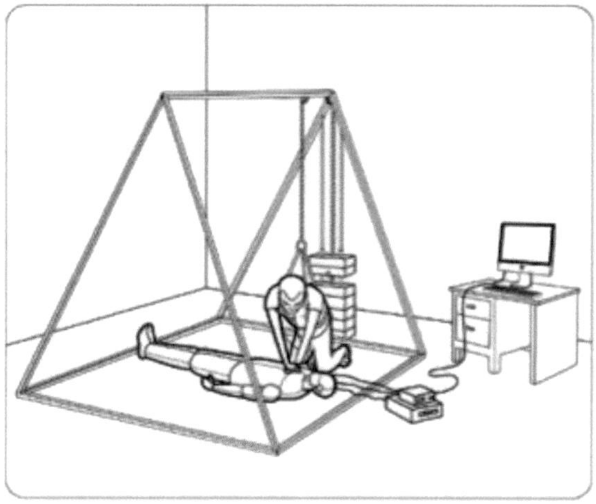

Figure 5. The body suspension device system of the MicroG Centre, with the CPR mannequin on the floor and volunteer assuming the terrestrial CPR position, being partially suspended through the counterweight system, simulating hypogravity.

For these ground-based hypogravity simulation studies, a standard CPR manikin (Resusci Anne Skill Reporter, Laerdal Medical Ltd., Orpington, UK) was modified to include a linear displacement transducer capable of measuring external chest compression (ECC) depth and rate. The steel spring located in the mannequin's chest depressed 1 mm with every 1 kg of weight applied to it. A real-time feedback of each ECC was provided to the volunteers via a modified electronic guiding system with an LED display. The LED display consisted of a series of coloured lights that indicated depth in mm of ECCs (red and yellow, too shallow; green, ideal). An ECC rate of 100–110 compressions/min^{-1} was established using an audio metronome. A 6 s interval between each ECC set represented the time taken for two mouth-to-mouth ventilations. Although not true to real life, by adding in these aids, it allowed standardisation of the volunteers as their experience and training in CPR varied.

3.1.2. *Parabolic flights*

Reduced gravity can be achieved with a number of technologies, each depending upon the act of free fall, such as drop towers, small rockets and parabolic flights. The latter is the only way to allow human subjects to be studied under conditions of microgravity or hypogravity. Therefore, many physiological and operational studies have been conducted by space agencies around the world in parabolic flights.

In parabolic flights, adapted airplanes execute a series of manoeuvres (parabolas), each providing around 20 s of reduced gravity (hypogravity) or weightlessness (microgravity), during which experiments can be performed and data collected. A typical NASA parabolic flight lasts 3 h and carries experiments and crewmembers. It climbs from an altitude of 7 km above sea level at a 45° (pull up) angle, traces a parabola (pushover) and then descends at 45° (pull out). Microgravity by means of free fall is experienced during the pushover phase. In the pull-up and pull-out segments, crew and experiments are subjected to hypergravity that ranges between 2 and 2.5 Gz [9].

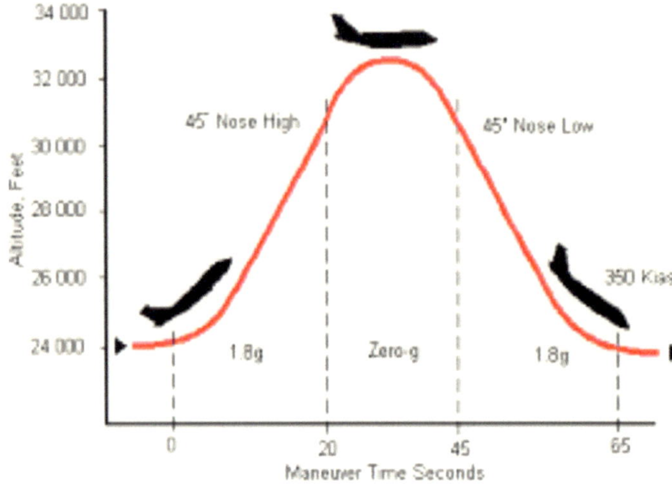

Figure 6. ESA parabolic flight profile, in which each parabola provides 20 s of microgravity that is preceded and succeeded by 20 s of hypergravity.

During a European Space Agency (ESA) campaign, there are typically 3 days of flights with 31 parabolas per flight. For each parabola, there are also two periods of increased gravity (approximately 1.8 Gz), which last for 20 s immediately before and after the 20 s of reduced gravity, as shown in **Figure 6**.

4. Extraterrestrial CPR methods

Some of the challenges faced in this unique environment have already been presented, including the practical, logistical and physical. The physiological changes and increased physical demands that occur in an extraterrestrial environment make the performance of CPR already difficult, but add to this, the limited storage and parameters found on any spacecraft or orbiting station, such as the ISS, and the task become all the more daunting, especially if ill prepared. To this end, several methods of CPR have been developed to bridge the gap between the time of occurrence of a cardiac arrest and the time when further resuscitation equipment can be available. These methods focus in particular on the ability of a single person to apply CPR, in particular the Evetts-Russomano (ER), reverse bear hug (RBH) and handstand (HS) CPR methods.

The rationale for the development of these single-person methods is that in microgravity, whether in a spacecraft or space station, all equipment is stored away as cabin space is limited and equipment floating freely is hazardous. Thus, the time to elapse between a fellow crewmember recognising the need for retrieval and deployment of life support equipment could range anywhere from 2 to 4 min [41]. This time period is obviously a critical window that will affect patient survival, and therefore, to maximise the chances of a successful outcome, a single-person method of microgravity CPR is needed so chest compressions can begin while advanced life support equipment is retrieved.

Evidence regarding the applicability and suitability of the three single-person rescuer methods discussed in the next section is scarce and varies for several reasons. Parabolic flights have been used to research these methods [4, 42, 43], and although these flights provide an excellent microgravity analogue, the short periods of actual microgravity provided mean the data collected and the conclusions drawn from the results have limitations. The majority of the scientific data comes from ground-based analogues, wherein these unique CPR methods can be studied over longer periods of time. Nonetheless, it is difficult with these analogues to fully reproduce the microgravity environment and physiological changes usually seen in microgravity. As with all analogues, they are good but never a perfect replication of the actual environment.

4.1. Evetts-Russomano CPR method

The ER technique is the newest of the three methods to be discussed and perhaps the most technically difficult, potentially requiring more training of the individual than other methods to ensure its proficient application. The rescuer places their left leg over the right shoulder of the patient and their right leg around the patient's torso, allowing their ankles to be crossed approximately in the centre of the patient's back; this is to provide stability and a solid platform against which to deliver force, without the patient being pushed away (**Figure 7(A)**). From this position, chest compressions can be performed while still retaining easy access to perform ventilation. When adopting the ER method, the rescuer must be situated in a manner that also allows sufficient space on the patient's chest for the correct positioning of their hands to deliver the chest compressions.

It is important to note that the rescuer simply wrapping their legs around the patient's waist is not an adequate position; this will not provide a firm enough base, and the chest compressions applied will extend the patient's back and reduce the actual depth of the compressions.

The advantage of the ER position over other methods is that by being face-to-face with the patient, single-person ventilation is easier. Initial parabolic flight and ground-based simulation data showed the ER method as delivering an adequate rate and depth of chest compressions, although this was according to the 2005 resuscitation guidelines [5, 42]. More recent data from ground-based simulations, using the updated 2010 guidelines, demonstrated that rescuers using the ER method fell slightly below par in terms of depth of compression but were able to maintain an adequate rate [45, 47].

A disadvantage of the ER method lies in its being technically more difficult and potentially requiring the most amount of training in order to be effective. In addition, the ER method is fatiguing after 2 min of chest compressions following the current guidelines, being considered more tiring than the HS method, although less so than the RBH technique. It has been found that rescuer fatigue leads to a failure to decompress the chest completely. This is a common problem across all three methods as fatigue takes effect, but it is more pronounced with the ER method, and this may be in part due to the positioning of the rescuer [48].

Although there is no statistical data to support the idea, it has been observed and surmised by researchers that height and anthropometric measurements may not be a predetermining factor for successful chest compressions using the ER method. This signifies that a rescuer

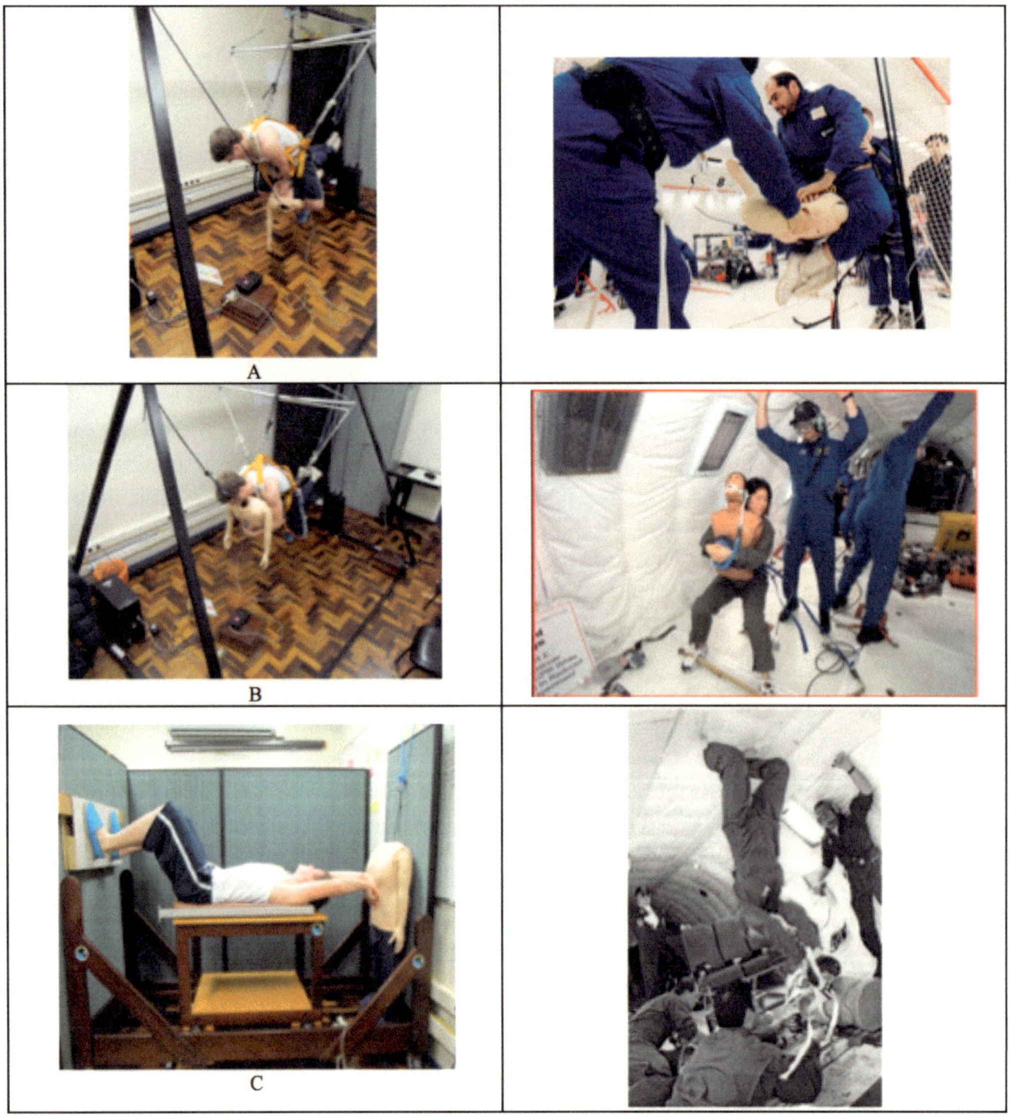

Figure 7. Three single-person microgravity CPR methods in ground-based microgravity simulations at the MicroG Centre and in parabolic flights: (A) Evetts-Russomano, (B) reverse bear hug and (C) handstand.

with short legs who may not be able to cross their ankles behind the patient's back may still be capable of performing CPR to an adequate standard using the ER method [5].

4.2. Reverse bear hug CPR method

The RBH method is possibly the simplest of the three single-person methods presented and is essentially similar to the Heimlich manoeuvre. The rescuer needs no additional equipment or to be wary of their surroundings as the RBH method is independent of capsule parameters.

The rescuer takes up position behind the patient to easily wrap their arms around the patient and lock their hands across the patient's chest. Arm flexion is primarily used to produce the force needed for chest compressions. The rescuer can use their legs to stabilise both themselves and the patient (**Figure 7(B)**).

The advantage of the RBH method lies in its simplicity to learn and apply. The rescuer can easily assume a position behind the patient, find the correct spot on the patient's chest and begin chest compressions. Parabolic flight data has shown the RBH method to be an effective method of CPR in simulated microgravity [4]. However, when assessed during a ground-based analogue over a prolonged period of time, such as 2 min, the RBH fell dramatically short of the current resuscitation guidelines [45]. Despite the relative simplicity of the method, ground-based studies suggest that it is an ineffective and inefficient method when performed over time. CPR using the RBH was seen to initially provide an adequate depth and rate of chest compression, in accordance with the most recent guidelines. Nonetheless, as early as the second cycle of chest compressions, rescuers rapidly tired—resulting in a decline in the depth of chest compressions and overall drop in the quality of CPR [44, 45]. Logistically, this method also presents a problem in ventilating as the rescuer is positioned to the rear of the patient. Assuming the rescuer is alone, they would need to rotate the patient so they are face to face in order to provide ventilations, before rotating the patient back again in order to continue compressions. This manoeuvring would delay the resumption of chest compressions and ultimately affect the quality of the CPR applied.

4.3. The handstand CPR method

Performance of the HS method also requires no equipment, but the patient does need to be placed against the inner side of the capsule or spacecraft in which they are located. Importantly, this must be a solid surface that is capable of withstanding the force and vibration generated by the application of the CPR. Once a suitable site to position the patient has been identified, the rescuer must then place their feet on the surface opposite to the patient, having their arms stretched out above their head, as demonstrated in **Figure 7(C)**.

From this position, the rescuer can flex/extend their hips while keeping their arms straight and locked on the patient's chest in the traditional spot, to generate the force needed for chest compressions. Parabolic flights [4] and ground-based simulations [45] have found the HS method to be the least fatiguing of the three single-person CPR methods, with rescuers able to provide an adequate depth and rate of chest compressions, in accordance with the latest guidelines [4, 44, 45].

The major limiting factor of this technique is its reliance on the physical parameters of the vessel itself. The HS method is dependent on a capsule that is between a range of diameters in order to have sufficient space for the patient and rescuer, as well as enough distance between the two to allow sufficient hip and knee movement in order to generate enough force for chest compressions. Furthermore, the height of the rescuer is crucial with this method; a shorter rescuer may not be able to achieve good placement of the feet on the surface opposite to the patient, thereby being unable to generate enough force and resulting in inadequate chest compressions.

4.4. Restrained CPR method: standard position

The restrained CPR method using the standard position is identical to that of terrestrial CPR but requires the use of equipment to restrain both the rescuer and the patient to prevent both from floating away from each other after the delivery of force. The restraint system currently used aboard the ISS is known as the crew medical restraint system (CMRS). The patient rests on the CMRS, which is used to strap the patient into a supine position. The standard technique, as the name suggests, is the same conventional CPR technique used on Earth. The difference lies in the rescuer having straps around their waist and a restraint cord across their lower legs (**Figure 8**). Researchers conducted in parabolic flights have shown this method to require a great deal of effort on the part of the rescuer, as they must counteract the force of the chest compressions. Thus, this method was seen to fatigue the rescuer quickly, even more so than the single-person HS method [4, 43].

4.5. Restrained CPR method: straddling position

In the straddling manoeuvre, the rescuer performs chest compressions by kneeling across the patient's waist but uses the same retraining equipment as with the standard technique. The delivery of the chest compressions is the same as that of terrestrial CPR, in that arms are kept straight and placed on the chest. The advantage of this position over the standard technique is that it requires less space. The standard position requires an area large enough for both the CMRS and rescuer to fit side by side, whereas the rescuer is positioned above the patient in the straddling technique, thereby reducing the total space in use. This could be an important factor to consider, given the limited dimensions of a spacecraft or the ISS. Despite the familiarity and

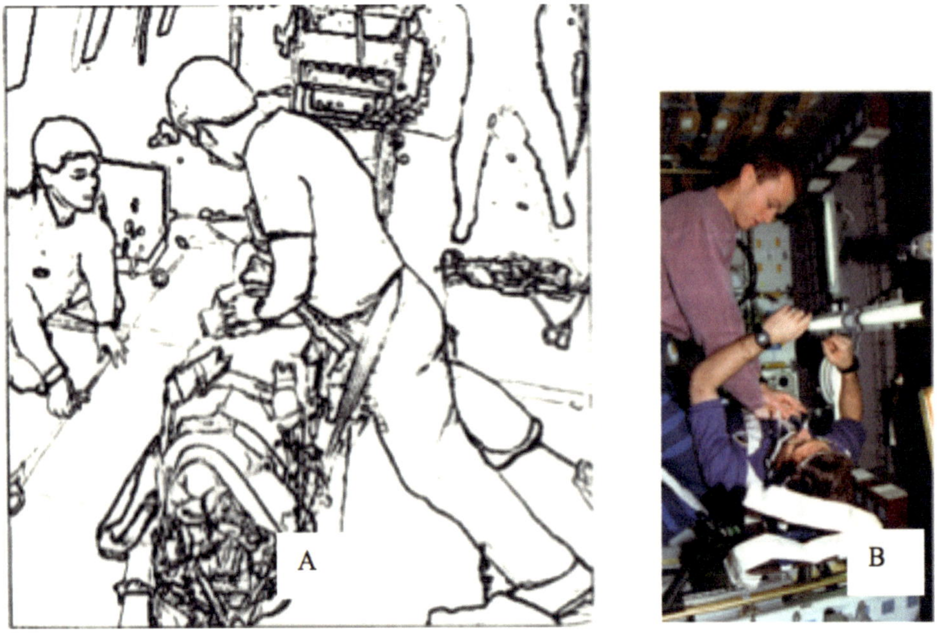

Figure 8. Crew medical restraint system (CMRS) being tested in a parabolic flight (A) and at the international space station (B) [43].

relative ease of use of these techniques, parabolic flight data has indicated that CPR performed using both restraint methods fall below current AHA guidelines, suggesting they may not be the most appropriate method to use in the event of a cardiac arrest scenario on board [43].

4.6. Hypogravity CPR methods

4.6.1. Terrestrial-style hypogravity CPR

In hypogravity, sufficient gravitational field is present on most celestial bodies that humans could encounter (Moon or Mars), meaning that CPR could begin without any adjuncts or equipment. Unlike the conditions for administering CPR in microgravity, the presence of at least some gravity in these environments makes CPR feasible with traditional terrestrial CPR. However, the technique of CPR may need adjustment to counter the negative impact of the reduced gravitational field. Traditional CPR instruction advises the use of straight, rigid arms placed on the patient's chest to perform compressions. However, a reduction in the upper body weight of the rescuer due to a reduced gravitational field will lead to a decreased ability to generate force through acceleration of the upper body and the subsequent transfer of that force through the straight arms. Research has shown that a natural tendency to adapt takes place, seeking to generate more force by flexing/extending the upper limbs in order to augment acceleration of the upper body [46]. In instances where traditional CPR in hypogravity is not sufficient to generate enough force to achieve the necessary depth of chest compressions, rescuers are encouraged to have a combined technique of accelerating their upper body and extending their upper limbs to generate enough force to compress the chest to 50–60 mm [45, 47].

4.6.2. The seated arm-lock (SeAL) method

The seated arm-lock (SeAL) method is a new concept but has many similarities to the traditional CPR technique used for hypogravity [49]. It was devised as a means of combatting the potential negative issues caused by performing CPR in hypogravity. The SeAL method involves the rescuer straddling the patient, with the patient's arms being locked in behind the rescuers' knees. The rescuers knees should be positioned in the shoulder area of the patient and their toes by the patient's hips (**Figure 9**). When used in a low-gravitational-field environment, the position prevents the rescuer from being pushed away from the patient by using the arms as a secure and comfortable pivot point. No residual tone is required in the patient's arms.

A small preliminary study found that rescuers were able to produce adequate depth of chest compression across a range of gravity conditions, Earth (1 Gz), Moon (0.38 Gz) and Mars (0.16 Gz). Additionally, the authors suggest that the SeAL method will allow the rescuer to be better secured to the patient and therefore prevent the two from being pushed apart from each other [49]. A preliminary study has recently been conducted at the MicroG-PUCRS, Brazil, testing a variation of this technique, called the Mackaill-Russomano hypoG CPR method. This adaptation of the SeAL technique sees the rescuer straddling the mannequin (CPR victim) and using their legs to embrace the legs of the dummy to act as an anchor. The weight of the mannequin legs were calculated and adapted to be in accordance with the gravitational force of the hypoG environment being simulated.

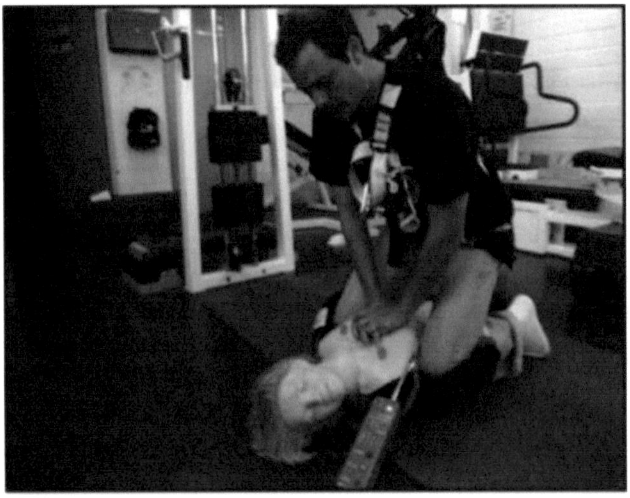

Figure 9. The seat arm-lock method in simulated hypogravity at the European Astronaut Centre.

5. Summary of ground-based space analogue studies

5.1. Microgravity CPR studies

Research into extraterrestrial CPR, particularly CPR in microgravity, has been ongoing for more than a decade. Several parabolic flight campaigns [4, 42, 43] have investigated the feasibility of the main CPR methods. As previously mentioned, although parabolic flights provide an excellent analogue of microgravity, their short duration (about 20 s per parabola) limits the amount of data that can be collected and interpreted. Accordingly, most of the available evidence investigating the different CPR methods has come from ground-based simulation studies, using such devices as the BSD. Although still with limitations, ground-based simulation studies do provide additional insight into the effectiveness and feasibility of microgravity CPR methods, particularly over prolonged time periods. Resuscitation guidelines are in general updated every 5 years, with adaptations made based on current evidence. This requires that CPR research in simulated extraterrestrial environments be periodically re-evaluated to determine if the various methods continue to meet current guidelines.

Earlier studies examining the ER method showed it could be administered and comply with the 2010 CPR guidelines while also correlating with parabolic flight data, indicating its use could provide effective CPR in microgravity. In addition, the research aimed to evaluate the physiological impact of performing the ER method, using subjective (Borg scale) and objective measurements (heart rate). Although found to be very tiring in comparison to terrestrial CPR, the ER method could be sustained effectively for up to 2 min [5]. Building on this work, comparative studies were conducted of the three main single-person CPR techniques, the ER, RBH and HS methods. A preliminary study comparing these methods proved the suitability of the BSD for conducting this type of research, which then led to a larger study. Results from the larger comparative study, carried out using the 2010 guidelines, found the HS method to be the most effective in terms of depth (also called 'true depth' to account for adequate decompression of the chest during ECC) and rate of administered ECCs, closely followed by the ER method, while the RBH gave the worst clinical results, as well as being extremely fatiguing (**Figures 10** and **11**). These studies also assessed the physiological cost of performing these methods, compared to terrestrial CPR. Using more objective measures, such as oxygen uptake (VO_2), these studies demonstrated that all three methods had a greater VO_2 than terrestrial CPR, with the HS being the least aerobically demanding and the RBH the most demanding [44, 48].

The physiological challenge of these methods is potentially a very important issue, as a well-documented decline in VO_{2max} occurs when in microgravity for a prolonged period, even when using countermeasures. These ground-based studies, which aim for 50–60 mm compression depth in accordance with both the 2010 and 2015 resuscitation guidelines, highlight the significant increase in VO_2 that takes place, when compared to the 2005 guidelines. These findings emphasise the importance of maintaining aerobic capacity in case the need to perform CPR in microgravity should arise [47, 50].

A series of studies have considered muscle activation, via superficial electromyography (EMG), while performing CPR in micro- and hypogravity, in order to understand the muscle groups used in comparison to terrestrial CPR. The rationale behind this was to potentially identify the responsible muscle groups so as to tailor exercise programs to ensure these muscle groups are maintained [6, 51, 52]. EMG data showed the triceps, pectoralis major and rectus abdominis muscles to be more active when conducting microgravity CPR, particularly for the ER method, when compared to 1 Gz and hypogravity CPR. This data adds to the evidence found in other studies indicating that astronauts need to maintain their muscle endurance in these particular muscle groups, as well as preserve their cardiorespiratory capacity to be able to adequately perform CPR should they need to in an emergency [52].

5.2. Hypogravity CPR studies

The BSD has also been successfully used in a series of studies evaluating CPR in simulated hypogravity. These studies have focused on the feasibility of performing CPR using the terrestrial method in hypogravity, as well as assessing the alterations in technique in hypogravity, physiological impact and weight as a pivotal factor in performing CPR in these environments. Initial hypogravity studies showed that CPR in hypogravity, particularly Lunar and Martian environments, was feasible using traditional terrestrial CPR. Furthermore, they highlighted the occurrence of an increase in the arm flexion angle of the rescuer [46]. Traditional teaching of BLS and CPR advocates that arms should be kept rigid in order to transfer the force of acceleration of the rescuers' upper body to the chest of the patient. These studies show that for CPR to be effective, and achieve guideline recommendations, the rescuer needs to flex and extend their arms, up to 14° (±8.1°), and use their upper limb musculature to generate force to compress the chest to a sufficient depth. This was even greater in microgravity using the ER method, up to 16.5° (±10.1°); however, as the technique used is markedly different to terrestrial CPR, a direct comparison between the two is difficult [46, 47, 50] (**Figure 12**).

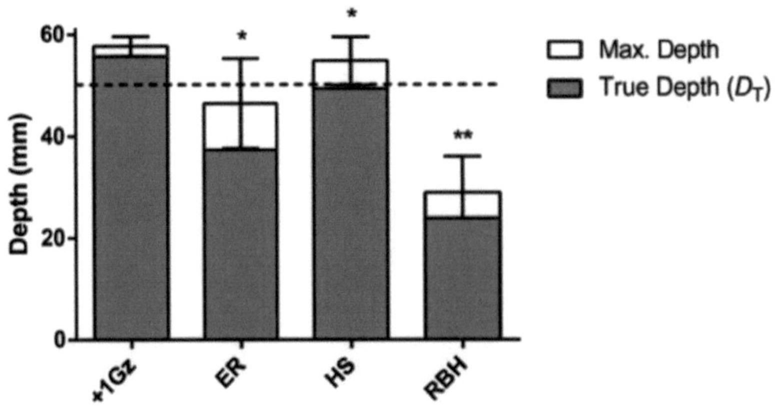

Figure 10. Mean true depth of ECC over 1.5 min for terrestrial and microgravity CPR using the three methods. Dashed line represents greater than 50 mm of depth set by the ILCOR 2010 guidelines; n = 23. Adapted from Ref. [48].

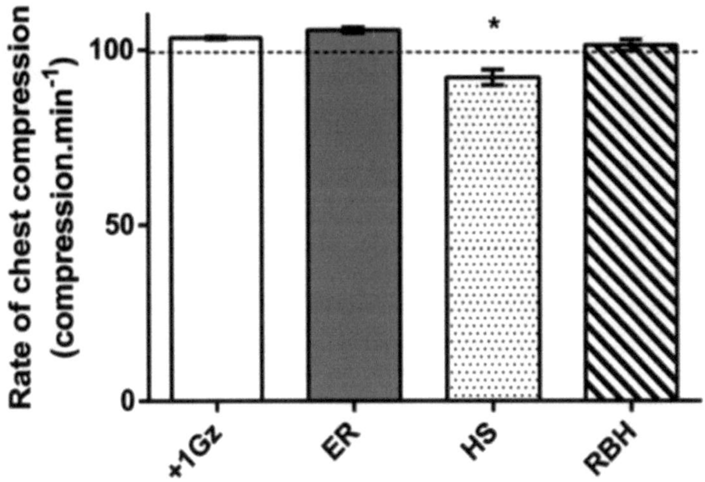

Figure 11. Mean rate of external chest compression (6 SEM) over 1.5 min for terrestrial and microgravity CPR using the three methods. Dashed line represents the lower limit of 100 compressions/min set by the ILCOR 2010 guidelines; n = 23. * Significantly different from +1 Gz, ER and RBH. Adapted from Ref. [48].

Similar to the microgravity studies, the physiological cost was measured subjectively and objectively, using the Borg scale and VO_2, respectively. Compared to terrestrial CPR, hypogravity CPR is more tiring and requires a greater VO_2, but not to the same extent as the microgravity CPR methods [47] (**Figure 13**). EMG hypogravity CPR studies have shown the occurrence of more muscle activation in the rectus abdominis compared to +1 Gz CPR, as the rescuer needs to accelerate their upper body faster to generate the same force as would be found at +1 Gz. Considering Newton's second law of motion, $F = m \times a$, a reduction in mass will require an increase in acceleration to maintain the same force.

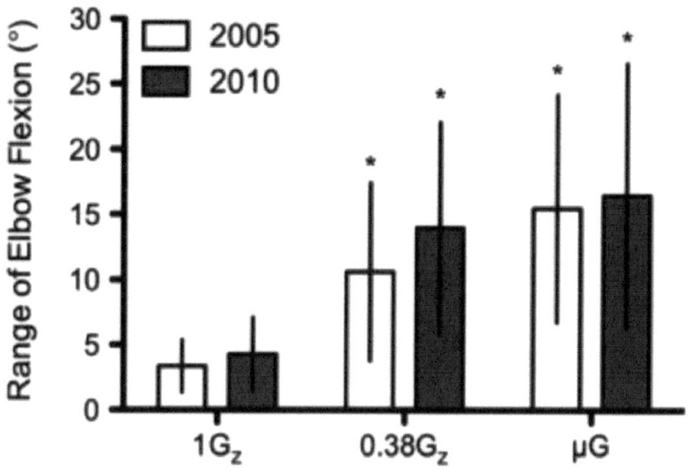

Figure 12. Mean (±SD) range of elbow flexion in the dominant arm at +1 Gz, 0.38 Gz and microgravity. Adapted from Ref. [47].

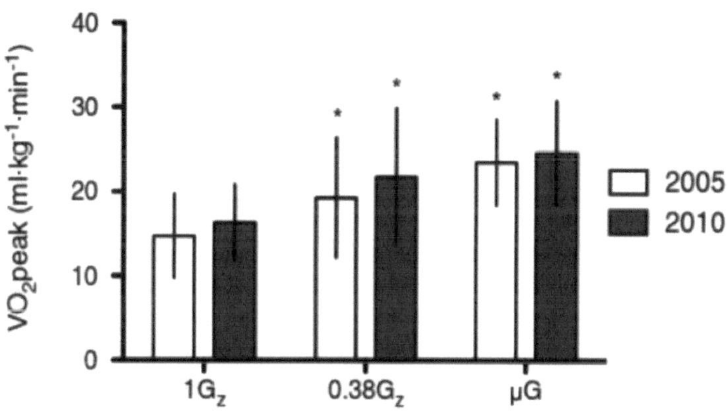

Figure 13. Peak oxygen consumption (VO_2peak) at +1 Gz, +0.38 Gz and microgravity.

Hypogravity studies have considered weight and gender and their importance in performing CPR in these reduced gravitational fields. As the data shows, the more you effectively reduce the rescuers' body weight or possibly muscle mass, the harder it is to generate force for ECC, and therefore the more tiring it becomes. As greater numbers of females join the astronaut corp, it is important to address the differences in weight and muscle mass to determine how pivotal they are in performing CPR in hypogravity. These studies demonstrated the possible existence of a gender difference in the effectiveness of BLS when delivering ECCs, according to the 2010 guidelines.

Female subjects were more likely to perform inadequate ECCs, as they tended to be shorter, weigh less and possibly have a smaller muscle mass than the males. Moreover, they were shown to have a higher physiological demand when performing ECCs. This was compared to males when performing CPR in hypogravity. Even when males had an effective reduction in their weight, they were still able to generate enough force to produce adequate depth and rate of ECC. This indicates that weight is not the only factor in effective ECC and that muscle mass may play an important role that counterbalances low-weight situations. Therefore, female rescuers may require additional strength training and alternative CPR techniques to overcome their lower bodyweight and muscle mass to ensure they can perform adequate ECCs in accordance with the current CPR guidelines [47, 50].

6. Extraterrestrial CPR guidelines

The extraterrestrial CPR guidelines presented in this chapter are based on the experience of the authors who conducted several studies at the MicroG-PUCRS, Brazil, and an extensive revision of the literature related to this topic. Therefore, the rationale behind specific guidelines for microgravity and hypogravity BLS and CPR is a combination of the novelty of the environment, increased physiological stress and isolated nature of these environments, all of which can affect the success of resuscitating a patient. However, familiarity and training of the appropriate BLS protocols and novel CPR methods for these environments will be a great benefit for both rescuer and patient. Furthermore, with the popularity of space tourism set to increase over the coming years, as private companies test new technology, there is a responsibility of space scientists and physicians to make sure that participants are familiar with and adequately trained in these novel BLS and CPR methods. Laypersons on Earth, such as schoolteachers and civil servants, learn BLS and CPR for a variety of reasons, and this custom should also apply to space tourists, who should be encouraged to become familiar with extraterrestrial resuscitation techniques. Therefore, extraterrestrial CPR guidelines have been developed and designed for all adults who will, for example, experience microgravity or hypogravity as part of their professional careers when participating in parabolic flights and space missions or who are involved in the training of astronauts.

Once cardiac arrest has been recognised, external chest compressions and ventilations need to be started immediately to maximise chances of survival. The best evidence for depth and rate of chest compressions come from international guidelines that are updated every 5 years by the International Liaison Committee on Resuscitation (ILCOR), who suggest changes to the European Resuscitation Council (ERC) and American Heart Association (AHA) based on the best possible evidence. Despite the well-documented altered physiology of astronauts in microgravity, there is insufficient evidence to suggest altering any of the parameters set by these international guidelines.

Summary of terrestrial ERC Guidelines for resuscitation (2015):

- Ratio of 30:2 (compression/ventilation).
- Rate of chest compression of 100 min^{-1} (but not exceeding 120 min^{-1}).
- Depth of chest compression between 5 and 6 cm.

- Ventilation should be 500–600 ml during CPR and given over 1 s; both breaths should take NO longer than 5 s to prevent interruptions to chest compressions.
- If there are more than one rescuer or ventilation equipment available, 10–12 breaths should be given every minute or one breath every 5 or 6 s, each delivered over 1 s. Observe for visible chest rise.

The specific guidelines for chest compressions in microgravity and hypogravity remain the same on Earth:

1. Compress the chest at a rate of 100–120 min^{-1}.
2. Each time compressions are resumed, place your hands without delay in the centre of the chest.
3. Pay attention to achieving the full compression depth of 5–6 cm (for an adult).
4. Allow the chest to recoil completely after each compression.
5. Take approximately the same amount of time for compression and relaxation.
6. Minimise interruptions in chest compressions.
7. Do not rely on a palpable carotid or femoral pulse as a gauge of effective arterial flow.
8. 'Compression rate' refers to the speed at which compressions are given, not the total number delivered in each minute. The number delivered is determined not only by the rate but also by the number of interruptions to open the airway, deliver rescue breaths and allow automatic external defibrillator (AED) analysis.

Chest compression-only CPR is important during resuscitation as it will benefit those who are not fully trained or are unwilling to perform mouth-to-mouth rescue breaths; this applies more to those who are entering hypogravity or microgravity as space tourists because all astronauts receive suitable BLS training. Under no circumstances should chest compressions be sacrificed for ventilations. Evidence suggests that compressions are more essential than ventilations during CPR and thus should be favoured during resuscitation [53]. There is no evidence to suggest that a change in ratio would be of benefit in hypogravity or microgravity. Therefore, rescuers should still aim for a ratio of 30:2 with a rate of compressions at 100 compressions min^{-1} and a depth of 5–6 cm, as stated above.

With regard to the depth of chest compression, it can be affected by the expansion of the chest in microgravity. There is no specific evidence to support changes to the terrestrial guidelines; however, it is theorised that a change in the chest wall dimensions of a patient in microgravity may alter the requirements for effective delivery of CPR, meaning that 5–6 cm may not be a sufficient depth of compression and a depth of >6 cm may need to be considered. However, more evidence is needed before contemplating any important change in these guidelines.

Currently, there is little supporting evidence for the best practice of ventilation in either hypogravity or microgravity. There is no reason to suppose that this would be different in a hypogravity environment, compared to terrestrial CPR. As the technique of CPR is essentially the same for both conditions, the rescuer should be equally capable of providing ventilations to the patient. The only caveat to this is if the patient and rescuer are in spacesuits, either while performing an extravehicular activity or walking on the surface of a planetary body, as the suit will obviously prevent them from giving mouth-to-mouth ventilation or administering CPR. However, future research into hypogravity BLS should evaluate the practicality of providing ventilations. With respect to microgravity, some research involving parabolic flight studies [4, 42] has evaluated ventilation, as well as chest compression depth and rate of these CPR methods. Findings have shown that rescuers using the Evetts-Russomano method were able to provide adequate ventilations of 491 ± 50.4 ml, in accordance to the 1998 ERC guidelines that applied at the time [42]. Other research focusing on the use of ventilation adjuncts, which required the mannequin to be intubated with a Kendall CardioVent device, showed that a lone rescuer could provide adequate chest compressions with the ventilation adjunct. However, setting up this equipment as a lone rescuer would delay the beginning of chest compressions and would go against the new guidelines, C-A-B, where compressions take priority [4].

Throughout these guidelines the patient refers to the individual who has a suspected cardiac arrest, and the rescuer refers to the person who is immediately responsible for their resuscitation. The initial sequence in determining if the patient is responsive remains very similar to the ERC 2015 CPR guidelines but takes into account the communication and resource limitations whenwnments (**Figure 14**):

- Check if you and other crewmembers are safe. If environmental factors are likely to be the precipitating factor (failure of life support systems, toxin build-up, trauma from projectile), make sure these are no longer a threat to you and other crewmembers before attempting to rescue the patient.
- Check for response—gently shake shoulders, and ask loudly in each ear, 'Can you hear me?' or 'Are you all right?'
- If patient does respond:
  - Find a suitable place to secure the patient to avoid risk of floating and suffering further trauma or leave them in their present position if no alternative is available.
  - Seek help from crewmembers, and attempt to determine what is wrong with the patient.
  - Reassess regularly until help arrives or communication is established with mission control/flight surgeon.
- If patient does not respond:
  - Shout for help immediately; when help arrives instruct them to find resuscitation equipment and more help. However, do not wait until they return; you must immediately begin chest compressions.
  - Follow the C-A-B sequence (compressions, airway, breathing).
  - Start chest compressions, selecting the appropriate CPR method depending on the environment you are in.

http://dx.doi.org/10.5772/intechopen.70221

- The lone rescuer should begin CPR with compressions rather than two ventilations to prevent any delay in giving the first compressions.
- Emphasis is placed on the lone rescuer beginning compressions before checking the airway, again to prevent any delay in chest compressions.

- If the patient is responsive and breathing normally:
  - Place in a safe position.
  - Send or call for help—call crewmembers or mission control.
  - Reassess the patient regularly.
- If they are not breathing:
  - Seek someone for further help, and establish communication with mission control. Further resuscitation and AED are required.

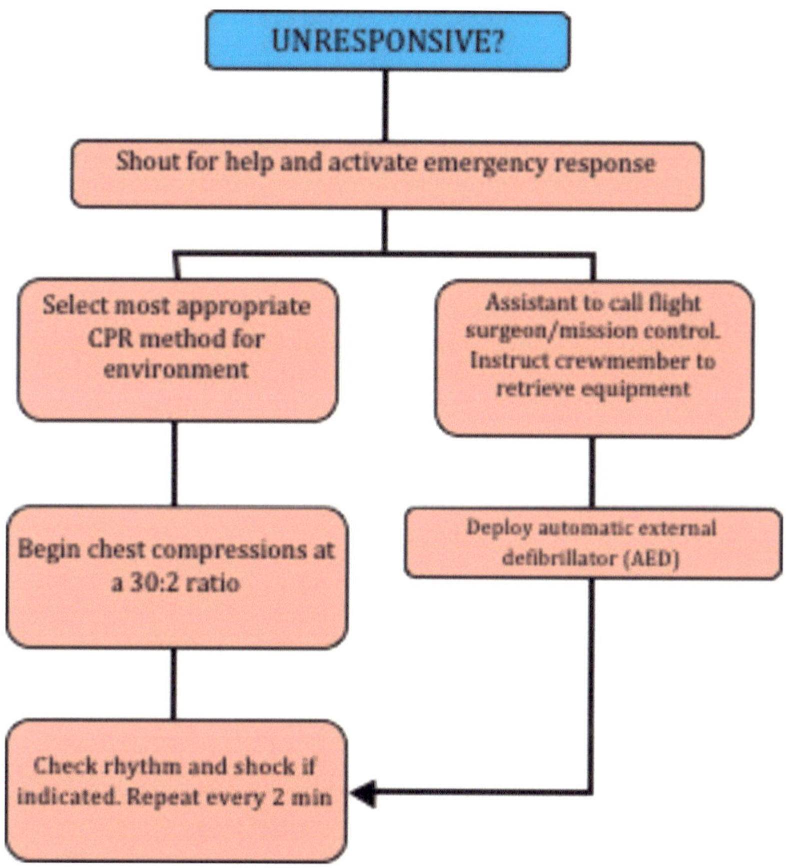

Figure 14. Microgravity and hypogravity adult basic life support algorithm, adapted from ERC 2010 guidelines. Reflect on the updated sequence of steps from airway, breathing and compressions (ABC) to compressions, airway and breathing (CAB).

- Start chest compressions, selecting the appropriate method depending on the environment you are in.

There is insufficient evidence, especially for the SeAL technique, to say which method is superior in hypogravity. However, it is recommended that the traditional terrestrial CPR method should be implemented first, as it produces adequate depth of compression with low levels of fatigue, suggesting that traditional CPR with an increased elbow flexion is an effective method of CPR [47]. **Figure 15** presents the algorithm for CPR to be applied in hypogravity environments.

6.1. Risks to rescuers

Altered physiology in microgravity and greater susceptibility to fatigue due to deconditioning could potentially affect the quality of CPR. The main factors that need to be considered are:

- Reduced gravitational field requires greater amount of force to be generated by the rescuer, resulting in increased muscle strain and shortness of breath in comparison to Earth.
- Deconditioning due to prolonged exposure to microgravity and/or hypogravity can place rescuers in a suboptimal physiological state when attempting to perform CPR. This could result in both a poor CPR performance and significant and rapid onset of fatigue.

Research examining CPR performance in simulated microgravity has shown all methods to be more fatiguing compared to terrestrial CPR [48]. CPR in hypogravity is also found to be more tiring than CPR on Earth, however, not to the same degree as in microgravity [47].

Current ERC guidelines recommend rotating rescuers every 2 min to prevent a drop in quality of chest compressions. A similar or possibly shorter window, such as 90 s, would be recommended for CPR in hypogravity. For microgravity, if enough crewmembers are present, an even shorter window for rotating is recommended, such as 60 s, to preserve the quality of chest compressions.

It is also important to consider that microgravity is a novel environment in itself and can be disorientating, which could be a potential hazard in an emergency scenario. The internal environment of a spacecraft or the ISS is also small, with confined spaces that can limit the ability of the rescuer and patient to manoeuvre and transfer during CPR or any emergency. Specifically for the HS method, particular consideration must be given to placement of the patient and positioning of the rescuer's feet, as lots of equipment are found within the capsule and there is the potential for damage to be caused to walls or partitions if they are not strong enough to withstand the force applied for performance of the CPR chest compressions. For the RBH and ER methods, there is always the danger of floating and hitting the sides of the internal environment of the capsule/spacecraft when performing CPR.

The use of an AED also imposes risks. Its use must be controlled and applied only by those trained to handle the equipment. Evidence shows that there have been few injuries due to poor AED use; however, the isolated and unique environment of microgravity in particular

http://dx.doi.org/10.5772/intechopen.70221

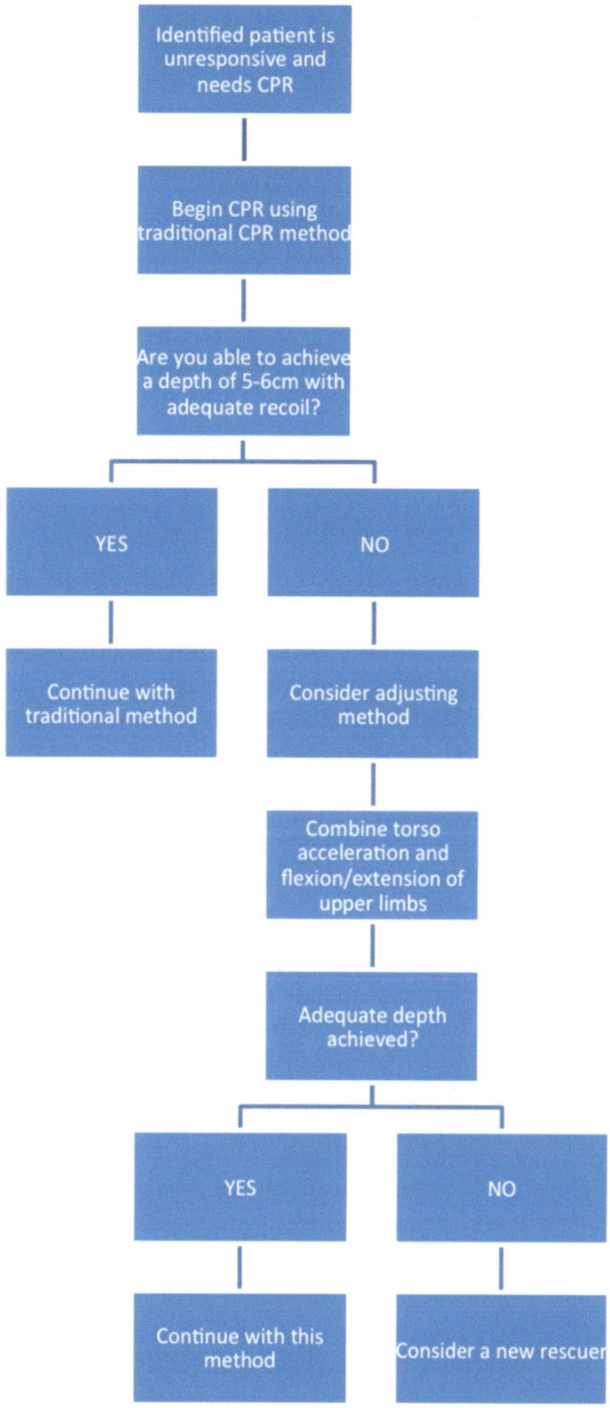

Figure 15. Algorithm for CPR in hypogravity.

can provide additional challenges in terms of making sure that rescuers are safe and clear when an AED is discharged.

7. Conclusion: extraterrestrial CPR—applications in space and on earth

As the space tourism industry commences and looks to expand over the following years, greater numbers of individuals will undertake suborbital flights and enter the microgravity environment. Before space tourism becomes a viable industry with regular flights, its technology will be tried and tested to the highest standards. The rapid rise in numbers of people who enter microgravity will pose a potentially significant increase in health problems, many of which participants will be unaware. Growing numbers of individuals will enter the space environment who will not have been subject to a strict preselection screening, such as that undergone by people preparing to join the astronaut corp [54]. This scenario could lead to potential difficulties: individuals will be at greater risk of a life-threatening cardiac event if they have not been screened for such health issues beforehand, and/or the physiological stress of launching and remaining in microgravity could exacerbate any underlying cardiovascular condition. This scenario could be further compounded by a shortage of individuals who have undertaken emergency training. This is a similar problem to that faced on Earth, with a varying uptake of BLS/CPR training across countries. However, the novelty factor of the microgravity environment combined with a serious medical emergency could create a highly stressful situation in which these bystanders are likely to be ill prepared and lacking the appropriate training necessary to carry out CPR techniques for the performance of adequate BLS. To this end, it is recommended that such individuals undergo appropriate training prior to a flight that would take them into an altered gravity environment. Healthcare professionals, schoolteachers and other civil servants who work with the public are currently given first aid and CPR training, and this exposure to basic BLS and CPR methods should be extended to all travellers into space. It is unrealistic to expect these individuals to be fully trained in all methods prior to launch, but familiarity with all methods, in accordance with ERC/AHA guidelines for CPR depth and rate of chest compressions, could better prepare them for the possibility of a serious cardiac event occurring that requires CPR.

Individuals who do find themselves in a situation of needing to administer BLS/CPR should initially follow the steps in **Figure 14**, making sure that a crewmember or ground control is aware that there is a medical emergency in progress. When commencing CPR, laypersons familiar with all three methods should be encouraged to perform the technique with which they feel the most comfortable and are consequently better able to deliver effective external chest compressions. As with the ERC/AHA guidelines, effective chest compressions should be favoured over ventilations.

Training and familiarisation with the novel CPR methods used in microgravity can enable laypersons to provide chest compressions and therefore maintain cardiac output and organ perfusion, until either a more qualified crewmember can takeover the procedure or until the craft ends its suborbital trajectory and returns to a normal gravitational environment where terrestrial CPR can commence. These steps will improve the chances of the patient having a favourable outcome.

Research into terrestrial CPR has shown that height and weight of the rescuer are correlated to effectiveness of chest compressions, and therefore, extraterrestrial CPR research could be used to improve terrestrial CPR, especially when physical disparities are encountered, such as when a rescuer is of smaller stature or lacks sufficient upper body weight. Examples of these scenarios include a child attempting to resuscitate an adult outside of a hospital situation or a small nurse resuscitating a large adult in hospital, who may also be obese or have significant lung pathology, such as pulmonary fibrosis or chronic obstructive pulmonary diseases, thus restricting further compliance of the chest.

Using the traditional straight-arm CPR technique, there reaches a point of critical mass when a rescuer is unable to overcome the resistance of the patient's chest to achieve the required 50–60 mm depth of chest compression. Without sufficient depth, not enough of a pressure gradient is created to circulate blood and perfuse organs. In these scenarios, the authors suggest a footnote to the CPR guidelines, concluding that extension of the upper limbs (triceps extension) can help augment the traditional straight-arm method with a synergistic acceleration of the body and extension of upper body to generate the force required to compress the chest.

Author details

Thais Russomano[1,2,3,4]* and Lucas Rehnberg[1,5]

*Address all correspondence to: thais.russomano@innovaspace.org

1 Centre of Human and Aerospace Physiological Sciences, Faculty of Life Sciences & Medicine, King's College, London, UK

2 International Space Medicine Consortium Inc., Washington, DC, USA

3 InnovaSpace Consultancy, London, UK

4 Human Spaceflight Capitalisation Office, Harwell, UK

5 University Hospital Southampton NHS Foundation Trust, UK

References

[1] Eisenberg MS, Horwood BT, Cummins RO, Reynolds-Haertle R, Hearne TR. Cardiac arrest and resuscitation: A tale of 29 cities. Annals of Emergency Medicine. 1990;**19**:179-186. DOI: 10.1016/S0196-0644(05)81805-0

[2] Baskett PJF. Peter Safar, the early years 1924-1961, the birth of CPR. Resuscitation. 2001;**50**:17-22. DOI: 10.1016/S0300-9572(01)00391-4

[3] Travers AH, Perkins GD, Berg RA, Castren M, Considine J, Escalante R, Gazmuri RJ, Koster RW, Lim SH, Nation KJ, Olasveengen TM, Sakamoto T, Sayre MR, Sierra A, Smyth MA, Stanton D, Vaillancourt C. Basic Life Support Chapter Collaborators. Part 3: Adult basic life support and automated external defibrillation: 2015 international

consensus on cardiopulmonary resuscitation and emergency cardiovascular care science with treatment recommendations. Circulation. 2015;**132**(16 Suppl 1):S51-S83. DOI: 10.1161/CIR.0000000000000272

[4] Jay GD, Lee P, Goldsmith H, Battat J, Maurer J, Suner S. CPR effectiveness in microgravity: Comparison of three positions and a mechanical device. Aviation, Space, and Environmental Medicine. 2003;**74**:1183-1189

[5] Rehnberg L, Russomano T, Falcão F, Campos F, Evetts SN. Evaluation of a novel basic life support method in simulated microgravity. Aviation, Space, and Environmental Medicine. 2011;**82**:104-110. DOI: 10.3357/ASEM.2856.2011

[6] Krygiel RG, Waye AB, Baptista RR, Heidner GS, Rehnberg L, Russomano T. The evaluation of upper body muscle activity during the performance of external chest compressions in simulated hypogravity. Life Sciences in Space Research (Amsterdam). 2014;**1**:60-66. DOI: 10.1016/j.lssr.2014.01.004

[7] Gell CF. Table of equivalents for acceleration terminology. Aviation Medicine. 1961; **32**:1109-1111

[8] Rainford DJ, Gradwell DP. Ernsting's Aviation Medicine. 4th ed. London: CRC Press; 2006. p. 800. DOI: 10.1201/b13238

[9] Barratt MR, Pool S. Principles of Clinical Medicine for Space Flight.1st ed. New York: Springer; 2008. p. 596. DOI: 10.1007/978-0-387-68164-1

[10] Alfrey CP. Effect of microgravity on the production of red blood cells. In: Research in the Microgravity Environment Related to Cardiovascular, Pulmonary, and Blood Functions and Diseases. Bethesda, MD: National Heart, Lung and Blood Institute and National Aeronautics and Space Administration Workshop; 20-21 January 1994. pp. 95-97

[11] Alfrey CP, Udden MM, Leach-Huntoon C, Driscoll T and Pickett MH. Control of red blood cell mass in spaceflight. Journal of Applied Physiology. 1996;**81**:98-104

[12] Riley DA, Ilyina-Kakueva EI, Ellis S, Bain JLW, Slocum GR, Sedlak FR. Skeletal muscle fiber, nerve, and blood vessel breakdown in space-flown rats. The FASEB Journal. 1990;**4**:84-91

[13] Riley DA, Ellis S, Giometti CS, Hoh JFY, Ilyina-Kakueva EI, Oganov V, Slocum GR, Bain JLW, Sedlak FR. Muscle sarcomere lesions and thrombosis after spaceflight and suspension unloading. Journal of Applied Physiology. 1992;**73**(2):33S-43S

[14] Oman CM, Lichtenberg BK, Money KE, McCoy RK. MIT/Canadian vestibular experiments on the Spacelab-1 Mission: 4. Space motion sickness: Symptoms, stimuli, and predictability. Experimental Brain Research. 1986;**64**(2):316-334. DOI: 10.1007/BF00237749

[15] Moore AD, Lee SMC, Stenger MB, Platts SH. Cardiovascular exercise in the U.S. space program: Past, present and future. Acta Astronautica. 2010;**66**(7-8):974-988. DOI: 10.1016/j.actaastro.2009.10.009

[16] Thornton WE, Hoffler GW, Rummel JA. Anthropometric changes and fluid shifts. In: Johnston RS, Dietlein LF, editors. Biomedical Results from Skylab. Washington, DC: NASA; 1977. pp. 330-338. (NASA Spec. Rep. SP-377)

[17] West JB. Historical perspectives: Physiology in microgravity. Journal of Applied Physiology. 2000;**89**:379-384

[18] Blomqvist CG, Stone HL. Cardiovascular adjustments to gravitational stress. In: Shepherd JT, Abboud FM, editors. Handbook of Physiology, Section 2: The Cardiovascular System, Vol III, Peripheral Circulation and Organ Blood Flow. Bethesda: American Physiological Society; 1983. pp. 1025-1063. DOI: 10.1002/cphy.cp020328

[19] Johnson PC, Driscoll TB, LeBlanc AD. Blood volume changes. In: Johnson RS, Dietlein LF, editors. Biomedical Results from Skylab. Washington, DC: NASA; 1977. pp. 235-241

[20] Fritsch-Yelle JM, Charles J, Jones MM, Wood ML. Microgravity decreases heart rate and arterial pressure in humans. Journal of Applied Physiology. 1996;**80**:910-914

[21] Charles JB, Lathers CM. Cardiovascular adaptation to space flight. The Journal of Clinical Pharmacology. 1991;**31**(10):1010-1023. DOI: 10.1002/j.1552-4604.1991.tb03665.x

[22] Shykoff BE, Farhi LE, Olszowka AJ, Pendergast DR, Rokitka MA, Eisenhardt CG, Morin RA. Cardiovascular response to submaximal exercise in sustained microgravity. Journal of Applied Physiology. 1996;**81**:26-32

[23] Levine BD, Lane LD, Watenpaugh DE, Gaffney FA, Buckey JC, Blomqvist CG. Maximal exercise performance after adaptation to microgravity. Journal of Applied Physiology. 1996;**81**:686-694

[24] Mader TH, Gibson CR, Pass AF, Kramer LA, Lee AG, Fogarty J, Tarver WJ, Dervay JP, Hamilton DR, Sargsyan A, Phillips JL, Tran D, Lipsky W, Choi J, Stern C, Kuyumjian R, Polk JD. Optic disc edema, globe flattening, choroidal folds, and hyperopic shifts observed in astronauts after long-duration space flight. Ophthalmology. 2011;**118**(10):2058-2069. DOI: 10.1016/j.ophtha.2011.06.021

[25] Alexander DJ, Gibson CR, Hamilton DR, Lee SMC, Mader TH, Otto C, Oubre CM, Pass AF, Platts SH, Scott JM, Smith SM, Stenger MB, Westby CM, Zanello SB. NASA Evidence Report: Risk of Spaceflight-Induced Intracranial Hypertension and Vision Alterations. 2012. Available from: http://humanresearchroadmap.nasa.gov/Evidence/reports/VIIP.pdf [Accessed: 14-03-2017]

[26] Johnston SL, Marshburn TH, Lindgren K. Predicted incidence of evacuation-level illness/injury during space station operation. Presented at the 71st Annual Scientific Meeting of the Aerospace Medical Association. Houston, Texas; 2000

[27] Calder A, Nijar J, Scarpa P. Use of ultrasound for diagnosis in microgravity: Comparative survey of NASA flight surgeon and consultant radiologist opinions. Aviation, Space and Environmental Medicine. 2007;**78**(3). p.134

[28] D'Aunno DS, Dougherty AH, DeBlock HF, Meck JV. Effect of short- and long-duration spaceflight on QTc intervals in healthy astronauts. American Journal of Cardiology. 2003;**91**:494-497. DOI: 10.1016/S0002-9149(02)03259-9

[29] Platts SH, Stenger MB, Phillips TR, Arzeno NM, Brown AK, Levin B, Summers R. NASA publication. Evidence based review: Risk of cardiac rhythm problems during space flight. 2010. Available from: https://ntrs.nasa.gov/archive/nasa/casi.ntrs.nasa.gov/20100017571.pdf [Accessed 14-03-2017]

[30] Fritsch-Yelle JM, Leuenberger UA, D'Aunno DS, Rossum AC, Brown TE, Wood ML, et al. An episode of ventricular tachycardia during long-duration spaceflight. American Journal of Cardiology. 1998;**81**:1391-1392. DOI: 10.1016/S0002-9149(98)00179-9

[31] Perhonen MA, Franco F, Lane LD, Buckey JC, Blomgvist CG, Zerwekh JE, Peshock RM, Weatherall PT, Levine BD. Cardiac atrophy after bed rest and spaceflight. Journal of Applied Physiology. 2001;**91**(2):645-653

[32] Huikuri HV, PekkaRaatikainen MJ, Moerch-Joergensen R, Hartikainen J, Virtanen V, Boland J, Anttonen O, Hoest N, Boersma LVA, Platou ES, Messier MD, Bloch-Thomsen P. Prediction of fatal or near-fatal cardiac arrhythmia events in patients with depressed left ventricular function after an acute myocardial infarction. European Heart Journal. 2009;**30**:689-698. DOI: 10.1093/eurheartj/ehn537

[33] Prisk GK. Microgravity. American Physiological Society. Comprehensive Physiology. 2011;**1**:485-497. DOI: 10.1002/cphy.c100014

[34] Paiva M, Verbanck S, Estenne M. Chest wall mechanics in microgravity: Results from parabolic flights. In: Proceedings of the 5th European Symposium On Life Sciences Research in Space; August 2003. ESA SP-336

[35] Elliot AR, Prisk GK, Guy HJB, West JB. Lung volumes during sustained microgravity on Spacelab SLS-1. Journal of Applied Physiology. 1994;**77**:2005-2014

[36] Prisk GK, Guy HJB, Elliot AR, West JB. Inhomogeneity of pulmonary perfusion during sustained microgravity on SLS-1. Journal of Applied Physiology. 1994;**76**(4):1730-1738

[37] Guy HJB, Prisk GK, Elliot AR, Deutschmann III RA, West JB. Inhomogeneity of pulmonary ventilation during sustained microgravity as determined by single-breath washout. Journal of Applied Physiology. 1994;**76**(4):1719-1729

[38] Vaida P, Kays C, Techoueyeres P, Lachaud JL, Riviere D. Pulmonary diffusing capacity and pulmonary capillary blood volume during parabolic flights. Aviation, Space, and Environmental Medicine. 1996;**67**:700 (Abstract 210)

[39] Prisk GK, Guy HJB, Elliot AR, Deutschmann III RA, West JB. Pulmonary diffusing capacity, capillary blood volume, and cardiac output during sustained microgravity on SLS-1. Journal of Applied Physiology. 1993;**75**(1):15-26

[40] Russomano T, Evetts SN, Castro J, dos Santos MA, Gavillon J, Azevedo DFG, Whittle J, Coats E, Ernsting J. A device for sampling arterialized earlobe blood in austere environments. Aviation, Space, and Environmental Medicine. 2006;**77**(4):453-455

[41] Hamilton DR. Personal communication 9 Sept 2004 - Current ISS Cardiac Arrest Procedures; 2004

[42] Evetts SN, Evetts LM, Russomano T, Castro JC, Ernsting J. Basic life support in microgravity: Evaluation of a novel method during parabolic flight. Aviation, Space, and Environmental Medicine. 2005;**76**:506-510

[43] Johnston SL, Campbell MR, Billica RD, Gilmore SM. Cardiopulmonary resuscitation in microgravity: Efficacy in the swine during parabolic flight. Aviation, Space, and Environmental Medicine. 2004;**75**:546

[44] Kordi M, Kluge N, Kloeckner M, Russomano T. Gender influence on the performance of chest compressions in simulated hypogravity and microgravity. Aviation, Space, and Environmental Medicine. 2012;**83**(7):643-648. DOI: 10.3357/ASEM.3171.2012

[45] Rehnberg L, Baers JH, Velho R, Cardoso RB, Ashcroft A, Baptista R, Russomano T. The pathway to new guidelines what can CPR in simulated hypogravity teach us about CPR on Earth? In: Proceedings of the European Resuscitation Council: Resuscitation 2014; 15-17 May 2014; Bilbao, Spain. Resuscitation; 2014. 85:S6

[46] Dalmarco G, Russomano T, Calder A, Falcao F, de Azevedo DFG, Sarkar S, Evetts S, Moniz S. Evaluation of external cardiac massage performance during hypogravity simulation. In: Wickramasinghe N, Geisler E, editors. Encyclopedia of Healthcare Information Systems. 1st ed. NY, USA: Medical Information science reference; 2008. Chapter E. pp. 551-560. DOI: 10.4018/978-1-59904-889-5.ch070

[47] Russomano T, Baers JH, Velho R, Cardoso RB, Ashcroft A, Rehnberg L, Gehrke RD, Dias MK, Baptista RR. A comparison between the 2010 and 2005 basic life support guidelines during simulated hypogravity and microgravity. Extreme Physiology and Medicine. 2013;**2**(1):11. DOI: 10.1186/2046-7648-2-11

[48] Rehnberg L, Ashcroft A, Baers JH, Campos F, Cardoso RB, Velho R, Gehrke RD, Dias MK, Baptista RR, Russomano T. Three methods of manual external chest compressions during microgravity simulation.Aviation, Space, and Environmental Medicine. 2014;**85**(7):687-693. DOI: 10.3357/ASEM.3854.2014

[49] Benyoucef Y, Keady T, Marwaha N. The seated arm-lock method: A new concept of basic life support in simulated hypogravity of the moon and mars. Journal of Space Safety Engineering. 2014;**1**(1):28-31. DOI: 10.1016/S2468-8967(16)30069-6

[50] Baers JH, Velho R, Ashcroft A, Rehnberg L, Baptista R, Russomano, T. Is weight a pivotal factor for the performance of external chest compressions on earth and in space? Journal of Exercise Physiology Online. 2016;**19**:1-15

[51] Waye A, Russomano T, Krygiel R, Susin TB, Baptista R, Rehnberg L, Heidner G, Campos F, Falcao, F. Evaluation of upper body muscle activity during cardiopulmonary resuscitation performance in simulated microgravity. Advances in Space Research. 2013;**52**:971-978. DOI: 10.1016/j.asr.2013.05.028

[52] Baptista RR, Susin TB, Dias MKP, Correa NK, Cardoso RB, Russomano T. Muscle activity during the performance of CPR in simulated microgravity and hypogravity. American Journal of Medical and Biological Research. 2015;**3**:82-87. DOI: 10.12691/ajmbr-3-4-1

[53] Hupfl M, Selig HF, Nagele P. Chest-compression-only versus standard cardiopulmonary resuscitation: A meta-analysis. Lancet. 2010;**376**(9752):1552-1557. DOI: 10.1016/S0140-6736(10)61454-7

[54] Rayman RB, Antuñano MJ, Garber MA, Hastings JD, Illig PA, Jordan JL, Landry RF, McMeekin RR, Northrup SE, Ruehle C, Saenger A, Schneider VS. Space passenger task force. Medical guidelines for space passengers. Aviation, Space, and Environmental Medicine. 2002;**73**(11):1132-1134

Chapter 9

Resuscitation of Overcooled Mammals without Rewarming

Kirill P. Ivanov

Additional information is available at the end of the chapter

http://dx.doi.org/10.5772/intechopen.68422

Abstract

Cold is a deadly danger for man. If the temperature of the surrounding air is +1°C, it is death for a naked man, owing to the arrest of respiration at the body temperature 25–28°C. After the heart is arrested, the death occurs at 23–24°C. Our aim was to prolong life at an absolutely deadly body temperature. This problem is important nowadays owing to a lot of sea catastrophes, the investigations in Arctic and Antarctic areas, and so on.

Keywords: rewarming, potassium ions, calcium ions, artificial ventilation

1. Introduction

Temperature is the most important criterion of life. As it increases, the limit is achieved quickly. For homoeothermic organisms, the body temperature between 42 and 45°C is practically incompatible with life. The cold diapason is substantially wider. Humans and mammals can decrease their body temperature to 32–33°C and then restore it without any pathological after effect. At lower temperature, rewarming becomes dangerous. A too intensive external rewarming results in increased oxygen consumption by various, almost indifferent, tissues, so that the brain and heart are subjected to a deficit in the energy material. In such a case, a deterioration of their functions occurs, which can result in the death of an organism. Generally speaking, the resistance to cold in living organisms is essentially higher than the resistance to heat. This is associated with the fact that a high temperature disrupts the tissues, whereas low temperature, to the contrary, favors the conservation of the tissue structure. According to the old data of Andjus [1], a rat frozen at 0 to −1°C revived for a short time if its heart was rewarmed by a special thermode, and thus its circulation was partially restored. However, rewarming a man at a very deep cooling is very dangerous since the distribution of temperature fields may appear unfavorable for the most important organs of a living organism: brain and heart. This can result in the death of deeply cooled organisms. But, let us consider the possibilities of resuscitation of overcooled organism by rewarming.

Rewarming is a conventional method of resuscitation of a frozen man or animal. However, this seemingly irreproachable procedure appears to require compliance with certain rules. First of all, the effect of rewarming the whole organism depends on the state of respiration and circulation. If these functions still operate at the temperature in the rectum 26–28°C, the rescue team has a hope to restore the organism's life. If a man's respiration is arrested upon deep cooling, but a weak circulation is still preserved, there is a hope for recovery of life, but it is very weak, since after arrest of respiration the heart operates briefly, by common opinion only for 15–30 min. Unfortunately, this period of time has not been adequately explored, and it is impossible to say something strictly definite about it. Burton and Edholm [2] described a case when a victim of cold lied in a cold morgue for several hours without respiration. He was supposed to have an extremely weak heart activity and eventually survived. It is supposed that only separate heart impulses remained in him, which resulted in a very weak circulation. It is conceivable that such cases are of frequent occurrences. In this instance, the absence of visual respiration is not the reason for sending a victim of overcooling to a morgue.

There is one more rule. During rewarming, if the brain is warmed more quickly than the heart, the supply of the blood to the brain may appear to be insufficient for the brain life and consequently for the life of the whole organism. At any rate, from the practical point of view, upon the arrest of respiration, the main emphasis must be placed on rewarming the heart. The attention must be focused on the problem that upon rewarming the whole organism, the brain was not rewarmed well before the heart [2–6].

Now we shall consider other methods, which can be used upon resuscitation of overcooled organism without general rewarming.

2. Materials and methods

The studies on the influence of the decrease in the content of potassium ions in the blood were performed on the isolated rat hearts. They were perfused by Krebs-Ginzelite solution with various concentrations of potassium, and the heart activity was studied at normal and decreased temperatures.

The experiments on the influence of calcium ion concentration in the blood on thermoregulation were carried out on white male Wistar rats 280–310 g in mass. After narcotization (125 mg of urethane per 100 g of weight intraperitoneally), the animals were fixed in a special stand. Polyethylene catheters were inserted into the femoral vein and artery for injections and for measuring the blood pressure. The temperature in the rectum (at a depth of 4.5 cm) and in the region of medulla oblongata was measured with the help of copper-constantan thermocouples. One hour after the beginning of narcotization and inserting catheters and thermocouples, the rat on a special stand was immersed into water with the temperature ~+8°C. In this case, the head and nostrils of the animal were located above the water level. The temperature of the animal body decreased gradually at a rate of about 0.35–0.40°C per minute. During the experiments, we periodically recorded the pneumogram (a carbon sensor on the animal breast) and electrocardiogram (ECG), and also measured the blood pressure in the femoral artery and the body temperature in the rectum and brain. The control animals were observed after the respiration arrest and immediately after injection of 1 ml of physiological solution as a placebo up to the moment of the heart arrest and the decrease in the arterial blood flow to zero. Another group of animals was injected with 1 ml of 0.5% solution of ethylenediaminetetraacetate (EDTA) into the femoral vein 8–10 min after the arrest of respiration.

Calcium ion concentration in the whole blood was determined by the method of direct potentiometry with film calcium selective electrodes. The method of determining Ca^{2+} concentration in the blood is described in detail in our previous work [5]. The blood samples for the determination of Ca^{2+} content had the volume not more than 0.3 ml.

We carried out the statistical treatment of the results with the help of Statistica program. We calculated the average values (M) and the error (m); the reliability of the differences was determined by Wilcoxson criteria (p_w).

Artificial ventilation was carried out with the help of special small self-made apparatus for the rats. The maximal power of the apparatus was 13–15 inhales per min. Each inhale contained 1.5 ml of air.

3. Results and discussion

3.1. Decrease in potassium ion concentration in the blood

A comparatively small increase in potassium ion concentration in the rat blood has no distinct effect on the thermal reactions of the animals. However, a decrease in the concentration of these ions in the blood upon its dilution results in a pronounced increase in the resistance to cold.

When an isolated heart of a rat is perfused with the blood with normal concentration of potassium ions (K^+ 5.9 mM), it terminates contractions as the temperature of the heart tissues decreases to 14–12°C. But if the content of K^+ in the blood with which the heart is perfused is 3.6 mM, the heart is arrested at lower temperature of about 10–8°C. If the K^+ content is reduced to 2.5 mM, a complete arrest of the heart will occur at 6–5°C (**Figure 1A–C**; **Table 1**) [7].

Therefore, a decrease in the concentration of potassium ions distinctly increases the heart's resistance to cold and, consequently, decreases the danger of disrupting the circulation. True enough, it is hardly possible to save the victim of overcooling at such low body temperatures with the help of decreasing potassium concentration in the blood. However, a dilution of the blood with the aim of decreasing K^+ concentration along with other procedures may be useful.

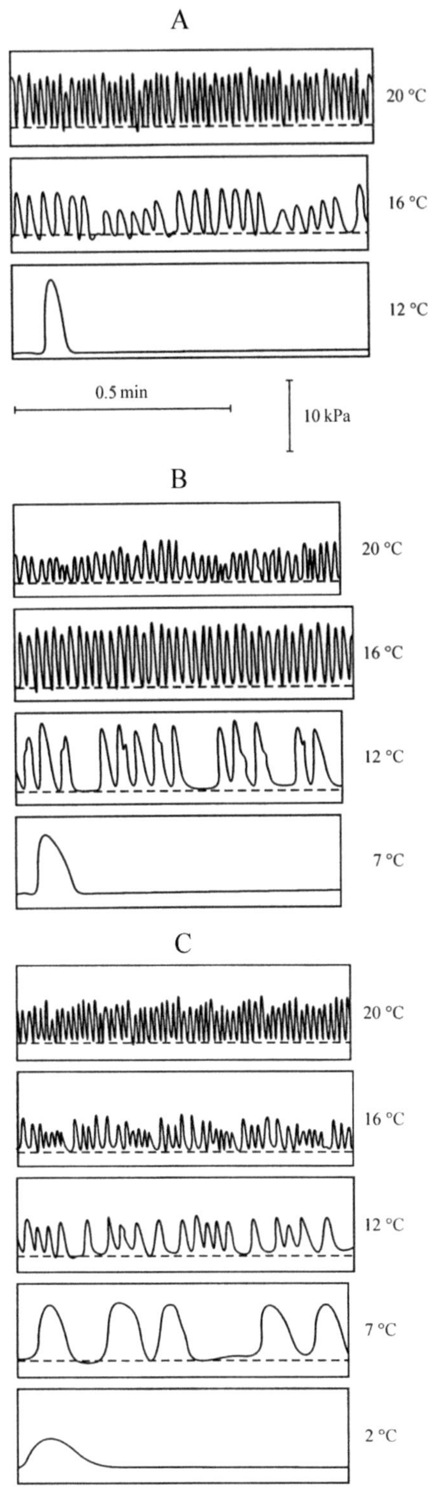

Figure 1. Mechanograms of the heart cooled and perfused with physiologic salt solution with K^+ content: (A) 5.9 mM; (B) 3.6 mM; (C) 2.48 mM.

Temperature of the hearts arrest, °C	
Perfusion with the solution with potassium content 5.9 mM	**After restoration of contractions by perfusing with potassium concentration 3.6 mM and further cooling**
14.2	9.8
12.0	7.5
12.9	10.2
15.0	12.0
11.7	8.3
13.2 ± 0.6	**9.5 ± 0.7**

Note: $P < 0.001$.

Table 1. Restoration of the contractions of cold paralyzed isolated hearts [6].

It appears difficult to find the data on the effect of ionic composition of the blood on their resistance to cold in the current literature. We were able to find a very interesting paper in Federation Proceedings [8], which supports our data about the role of potassium in this process. Furthermore, the effect of a decrease in potassium concentration on the increase in the heart tissues resistance to cold is very interesting and important from theoretical point of view. We emphasize that this fact opens the way to the studies of a number of other ions with the same purpose. The mechanisms of such action of ions are very interesting; however, such investigations seem to be scarce in the current literature.

3.2. Decrease in calcium ion concentration in the blood

As far back as in 1986, Hochachka [9] reported that in an overcooled organism, the cells die owing to the excess of calcium ions resulting from disrupting metabolism. These extra calcium ions must be removed from the intercellular fluids, but this process requires energy. The matter is that the concentration of calcium ions in the cells is about 10^{-8} M and in the intercellular fluids it is 10^{-3} M, thus we have the diffusion against a great concentration gradient, and the energy deficit in an overcooled organism prevents it.

We decided to examine the effect of calcium ion concentration in the blood on resuscitation of the functions of an overcooled organism.

We did not find any essential changes in the thermoregulation upon a small increase in the Ca^{2+} concentration in the blood. However, when the most important thermoregulation reaction—the cold shivering—is completely oppressed upon deep cooling of an organism, a comparatively small decrease in calcium ion concentration restores this most important muscle reaction in a short period of time (**Figure 2**) [5]. At a low body temperature of an animal, it is recommenced if a solution of ethylenediaminetetraacetate (EDTA) is introduced into the blood. EDTA decreases the calcium ion concentration since it reacts with them to give a complex compound, thus practically removing them from the blood. The introduction of 1 ml of 0.5% solution of EDTA into the blood of a rat 210–240 g in mass results in a decrease in calcium ion concentration by 15–25%. We emphasize that EDTA is a pharmacological preparation which is in wide use in medicine, and we inserted it in the relationships never exceeding those recommended for animals and humans.

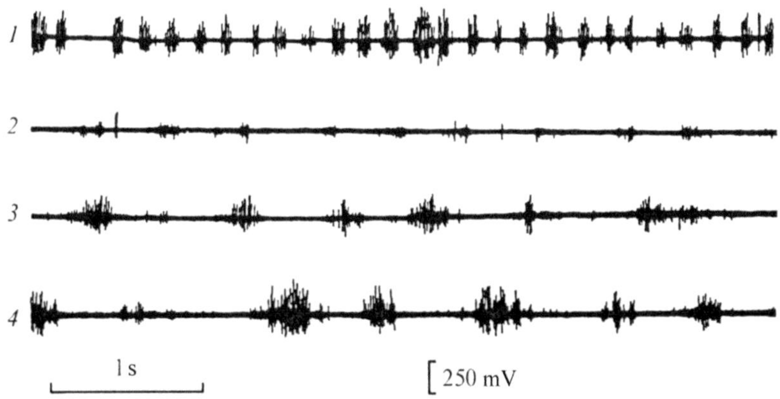

Figure 2. Arrest of cold shivering and thermoregulation tone in rats during cooling of the body and restoration of these physiological functions without rewarming the body after inserting 0.016 mmol of EDTA into the blood. (1) Brain temperature (Tb)—28°C; rectum temperature (Tr)—25°C; maximal intensity of the cold shivering and of the thermoregulation muscle tone. (2) Tb—20°C; Tr—17.2°C; retardation of the functions of thermoregulation center and an almost complete oppression of shivering. (3) Five min after inserting 0.016 mmol of EDTA into the blood: Tb—18.9°C, Tr—17.2°C. (4) Ten min after a repeated insertion of the same dose of EDTA (0.016 mmol): Tb—18.7°C, Tr—17.2°C.

If a decrease in calcium ion concentration exhibits such a distinct positive effect on the most important thermoregulation reaction, the question arises inevitably about how such an action will influence respiration, heart activity, and blood pressure at a low body temperature.

Tables 2 and **3** [10] answer this question. According to these data, EDTA excites the cold paralyzed respiration center and makes it work at a temperature, which under normal conditions results in its cold paralysis. Moreover, a partial restoration of the work of respiration center after EDTA insertion not only restores the cold shivering but also increases the frequency of the heart contractions and the blood pressure. Even though all these functions appear in an abruptly slowed down rhythm, this effect may continue for 1–1.5 h. Only gradually, it tapers down to nothing. If the cooling is stopped, and the animals are removed from water, dried, and left at room temperature, in this case the animal is warmed up on its own during 2.5–3 h

Temperature in the rectum, °C	Temperature in the brain, °C	Arterial blood pressure, mm Hg	Respiration frequency, cycles/min	Frequency of the heart contractions, imp/min
13.5	13.9	20	0	25
11.4	13.4	10	0	10
12.8	14.0	18	0	25
14.0	15.0	10	0	10
13.2	15.7	18	0	20
14.3	16.1	10	0	19
14.8	15.8	24	0	16
13.4 ± 0.6	**14.8 ± 0.2**	**16 ± 6.1**	**0**	**21 ± 5.0**

Table 2. Physiological parameters of the rats in 15 min after the arrest of respiration.

Temperature in the rectum, °C	Temperature in the brain, °C	Arterial blood pressure, mm Hg	Respiration frequency, cycles/min	Frequency of the heart contractions, imp/min
11.6	13.8	36	6	41
12.3	13.8	48	8	84
13.2	15.6	66	24	63
14.1	15.6	50	18	66
9.5	14.9	24	6	36
12.7	15.4	36	12	52
12.2 ± 0.7	**14.9 ± 0.3**	**43 ± 6.**	**12 ± 6**	**57 ± 7**

Table 3. Physiological parameters of these very animals after the arrest of respiration and immediate insertion of 1 ml of 0.5% EDTA solution into the blood.

and later does not differ from other control rats by its behavior. In this case, the insertion of EDTA saves the animal from death.

If a comparatively small decrease in calcium ion concentration exerts such an effect on an animal, it is necessary to reveal the action of this factor on the whole thermoregulation system, that is, on peripheral and central thermosensors. First, we tried to reveal the effect of a decrease in calcium ion concentration by 15–20–25% on the skin thermoreceptors. These experiments were carried out on the skin thermoreceptors of the nose and back skin of a rabbit. They were rather complicated since we have not always met with success trying to keep the even pulsation of the cold thermoreceptors for 1–2 h in the starting state before cooling and then for a sufficiently long time after cooling and EDTA insertion. In **Table 4**, we demonstrate five experiments which distinctly show the restoration of receptor pulsation after their cold paralysis in several minutes after insertion of EDTA solution into the blood [10]. The restored pulsation after its complete or partial oppression with cold continues variously from 20 to 30 min and even more. The secondary paralysis may result from restoration of calcium ion concentration in the blood to the norm.

Number of receptor	Skin temperature at the site of receptor location, °C	Pulsing frequency before EDTA insertion, imp/s	Maximal pulsing frequency after EDTA insertion, imp/s	Skin temperature in the same site of receptor location, °C
1	5.0	0	18	5.0
2	3.0	3	18	3.0
3	0	0	16	0
4	4.8	0	20	4.0
5	0	3	11	0
Mean ± SEM	**2.6 ± 3**	**1 ± 1**	**17 ± 2**	**2.4 ± 3**

Table 4. Pulsing frequency of thermoreceptors in 5–10 min after EDTA insertion at the skin temperature at the site of their location from 0 to +5°C.

Of course, it was of great interest and importance from theoretical and practical point of view to learn how a decrease in calcium ion concentration affects the center of thermoregulation apparatus immediately. The neurons taking part in thermoregulation are known to be located in various parts of the central nervous system, in the hypothalamus among them. Hence, in order to put the central nervous thermoregulation as a whole to a test, we decided to insert EDTA immediately into the brain ventricles of the animals. We selected a minimal dose of 10–15 mmoles for the whole rate 210–240 g in mass. This dose is many times less than the dose that had been inserted into the blood of these animals. As has been found earlier, respiration is completely paralyzed at the rat body temperature 17–18°C. The insertion of this dose of EDTA into the brain ventricles restored the respiration in its frequency and amplitude in 10–15 min, though still far from the norm, that is, the respiration center acquired a certain resistance to cold. Later, we carried out many experiments and confirmed all the results [6]. That means an inhibiting effect of cold on thermoregulation, respiration, and circulation and removal of the cold paralysis from these functions at the expense of activation of peripheral and central thermosensors.

3.3. Artificial ventilation

This is another method of saving a man from death during hypothermia.

Usually, artificial ventilation is considered as a help for the lungs in supplying an organism with oxygen. This is so indeed. A conventional artificial ventilation by manual operation without a special device may appear low efficient and give no expected result for 1 or even 2 h of its use even if there is a weak circulation.

It is seen from **Tables 5** and **6** that the lung respiration disappeared in the animals at the temperatures in the rectum 15.4°C, in the esophagus 16.6°C, in the brain 17.9°C (**Table 5**). In 12–15 min, when the temperature decreased by 1.5–2.0°C more, we switched on the artificial

Temperature in the rectum, °C	Temperature in the esophagus, °C	Temperature in the brain, °C	Respiration frequency, cycles/min	Frequency of the heart contractions, imp/min	Arterial blood pressure, mm Hg
15	16	17.6	0	17	25
17.2	18.4	19.7	0	21	20
14	15	16.3	0	17	30
14.5	15.3	16.6	0	23	10
15.5	17.4	18.7	0	24	24
14.5	15.8	17.1	0	28	18
17	18.4	19.3	0	19	14
15.4 ± 0.5	**16.6 ± 0.5**	**17.9 ± 0.5**	**0**	**21.3 ± 1.5**	**20.4 ± 2.6**

Table 5. Arrest of respiration and an abrupt decrease in the arterial blood pressure and in the frequency of the heart contractions after the animals stay in water with the temperature 8–9°C.

Temperature in the rectum, °C	Temperature in the esophagus, °C	Temperature in the brain, °C	Respiration frequency, cycles/min	Frequency of the heart contractions, imp/min	Arterial blood pressure, mm Hg
13.7	14.9	16.4	13	58	40
14	15.2	17	13	45	30
13	14.4	15.6	12	55	46
13.9	14.8	15.8	12	58	28
13.9	15.9	17.6	12	72	42
12.5	14.4	15.6	12	44	36
14.5	15.6	17.0	12	70	40
13.6 ± 0.2	**15.0 ± 0.2**	**16.4 ± 0.3**	**12.3 ± 0.2**	**57.4 ± 4.1**	**37.4 ± 2.5**

Table 6. Test rats 2 min after starting artificial respiration of 12–13 inhales per min.

ventilation. Two min after switching on the artificial ventilation, as is seen from **Table 6**, a distinct increase in the frequency of the heart contractions and in the blood pressure occurred, which is necessary for increasing the muscle heat production. If at this point we stopped cooling the animal, that is, removed it from cold water, artificial ventilation resulted in further increase in the frequency of the heart contractions and in the blood pressure, and in 2.5–3.5 h the animal restored completely the normal frequency of the heart contractions and the normal frequency of respiration and arterial blood pressure. But if the artificial ventilation was absent, at this low body temperature, the heart work gradually slowed down, oxygen consumption decreased, and the blood pressure decreased to zero. The animal died.

3.4. The last reserve for saving a homoeothermic organism from cold

Up to 0°C cold does not destroy the construction of the tissues. Consequently, no mechanical destructions of the tissues occur in the death from cold. In a complete physiological rest, the organism tissues consume a physiological minimum of energy. In a man of average weight and age, the energy consumption on the level of normal metabolism is about 1860 kcal per day. This is the required level of energy for maintaining all the living processes in various organs and tissues of a man at a relative rest. If a man is cooled and his average body temperature decreases, the energy consumption also decreases naturally. If a decrease in the energy supply of the tissues appears to be lower than the required quantity, under specific conditions, the tissues die. The last reserve for maintaining the living ability of the tissue is the limit of its temperature decrease (up to 0°C) and the limit of the decrease in the oxygen consumption. With the aim of preventing the animal brain from being devoid of the blood influx and of the minimum of oxygen, we slightly warmed up the heart to 19–20°C. Under these conditions, the heart retained its living ability and provided the brain with a minimum of oxygen and energy at its temperature of about 0°C. This means that under a sufficiently slow and careful rewarming, the heart, the brain, and the organism as a whole can still return to life. **Figure 3** shows one of the experiments of this series. As can be seen from the figure, the brain, after the

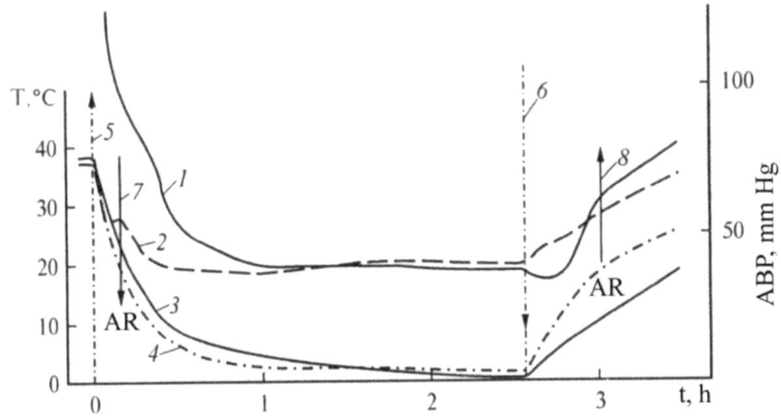

Figure 3. Cooling the rat brain to 1°C under artificial respiration, and local warming the heart retaining the arterial blood pressure at the level 40–45 mm Hg. *X*-axis—the time, h. *Y*-axis to the left—the temperature in the brain and in the rectum; to the right—arterial blood pressure, mm Hg. (1) Arterial blood pressure; (2) t° of the heart; (3) t° in the rectum; (4) t° in the brain; (5) the beginning of cooling the animal; (6) the beginning of warming up; (7) switching on the artificial respiration; (8) switching off the artificial respiration.

beginning of cooling, retained the temperature close to 0°C for a period of about 1.5 h. After the beginning of a careful rewarming, the brain temperature started to increase rapidly, and so did the arterial blood pressure. This experiment showed that the brain retained its living ability and still could exert control over the circulation being at a temperature close to 0°C for about an hour and a half. These animals after a complete resuscitation did not differ in anything from the control rats. This is a very important fact both for the theory of living activity of various animals and from the point of view of practical medicine. This supports the old observations of Andjus on overcooled rats [1]. Now we know that a severe minimum of metabolism is retained up to the lowest temperatures of about −100 or −130°C [11]. At such temperatures, the tissues acquire a complete independence from further decreases in temperature, since they have no need in energy anymore and pass into "eternal" existence without energy.

4. Conclusions

In this short chapter, we gave several sufficiently impressive remarks about the physiological mechanisms of the death and physiological mechanisms of resuscitation of mammals and humans during deathly hypothermia. As has been noted, cold does not destroy the construction of tissues. Ultimately, it only denudes the tissues of oxygen. According to a known axiom, only oxygen releases energy necessary for the living activity of all the organs and tissues as the result of oxidation reactions with carbohydrates, fats, and proteins. There is no alternative to oxygen. Therefore, hypoxia and cold are almost to the same extent responsible for the result and for resuscitation during hypothermia. This is an important reasoning. We hope that medicine will estimate it highly enough and will use it.

In practical medicine, the arrest of respiration and an abrupt decrease in the body temperature are the reasons for sending the "corps" to a morgue. Our experiments show that there are many prerequisites for resuscitation of the victim of overcooling. We suggest that this property of a living material to retain the living ability during a complete loss of the main life symptoms will make possible for the future science the creation of a living creature, which would lose life for centuries and recover after this great period of time. Broadly speaking, the conservation of life with cold is a large and badly developed problem. Of course, for the complete success of this act, a hard and long work is necessary, in the first place the study of the mechanisms of heat production in mammals and the reasons for its decrease up to a complete arrest. The latter is the main trend of our studies.

Author details

Kirill P. Ivanov

Address all correspondence to: kpivanov@nc2490.spb.edu

Laboratory for Physiology of Thermoregulation and Bioenergetics, I.P. Pavlov Institute of Physiology, Russian Academy of Sciences, St. Petersburg, Russia

References

[1] Andjus RK. Suspended animation in cooled, supercooled, and frozen rats. Journal of Physiology (London). 1955;**128**(3):251-254

[2] Burton AC, Edholm OG. Man in Cold Environment. London: Arnold; 1955. p. 333

[3] Alyukhin YS. Mechanics and energetics of the heart upon progressing hypothermia. I. M. Sechenov Physiological Journal. 1992;**78**(12):132-140

[4] Alyukhin YS. Functional activity, energetics, and surviving of the heart under hypothermia. Uspekhi Sovremennoi Fisiologii. 1998;**29**(3):66-78

[5] Ivanov KP. Principles of Energetics in an Organism: Theoretical and Applied Aspects. Vol. 3. St. Petersburg: Nauka; 2001. p. 277 [In Russian]

[6] Ivanov KP. Principles of Energetics in an Organism: Theoretical and Applied Aspects. Vol.4. St. Petersburg: Nauka; 2004. p. 252 [In Russian]

[7] Alyukhin YS, Ivanov KP. Increase in the resistance to cold of isolated rat heart after cold arrest without rewarming. Doklady Akademii Nauk SSSR. 2002;**386**(6):832-834

[8] Angelacos E, Maher J, Burlington R. Spontaneous cardiac activity at low temperatures. Federation Proceedings. 1969;**28**(3):1216-1219

[9] Hochachka PW. Different strategies against hypoxia and hypothermia. Science. 1986;**231**:234-241

[10] Ivanov KP. Resuscitation of vital activity after cold arrest of respiration by physiological methods without rewarming the body. Vestnik Rossiiskoi Akademii Meditsinskikh Nauk – Annals of Russian Academy of Medical Sciences. 2014;**7-8**:5-9

[11] Lozino-Lozinskii LK. Essay About Criobiology. Leningrad: Nauka; 1972. p. 280 [In Russian]

Chapter 10

Strategies of Neuroprotection after Successful Resuscitation

Enikő Kovács and Endre Zima

Additional information is available at the end of the chapter

http://dx.doi.org/10.5772/intechopen.70593

Abstract

Post-cardiac arrest syndrome (PCAS) incorporates post-cardiac arrest brain injury, post-cardiac arrest myocardial dysfunction, systemic ischemia/reperfusion syndrome and the precipitating pathology. Brain injury remains the leading cause of death in the post-cardiac arrest period. One of our main goals during post-resuscitation care is to guide a proper neuroprotective strategy. We are going to summarize the tools of neuroprotection in post-cardiac arrest therapy. The role of normoxia/normocapnia, normoglycemia, seizure control, sedation and pharmacologic strategies will be discussed in brief. The handling of temperature management and the management of hemodynamic variables to secure satisfactory cerebral perfusion will be worked out in details. Targeted temperature management is the main tool of neuroprotection in post-cardiac arrest therapy. We are going to conclude the principles of temperature control after successful resuscitation pointing out its beneficial effects. This method has also several complications that are going to be discussed highlighting its hemodynamic impacts. There is no evidence about target hemodynamic parameters during post-cardiac arrest syndrome to maintain cerebral perfusion neither about the most effective hemodynamic monitoring system. We are presenting preliminary data of our study where we investigate the effect of PiCCO™ (Pulse index Continous Cardiac Output) monitoring on the outcome in this patient group.

Keywords: post-cardiac arrest syndrome, post-cardiac arrest brain injury, post-resuscitation therapy, targeted temperature management, hemodynamic parameters

1. Introduction

Sudden cardiac arrest is one of the leading causes of death in Europe [1]. The outcome is still very poor: the hospital discharge varies between 7 and 10% after out-of-hospital cardiac arrest (OHCA) and it is approximately 25% after in-hospital cardiac arrest (IHCA) [1]. The chain of survival describes links that lead to a successful resuscitation [2]. The fourth element covers proper post-resuscitation care to restore quality of life. It is well known that the management of post-resuscitation cardiac arrest syndrome affects outcome and it is an important part of the resuscitation process. Pointing out the growing importance of post-resuscitation therapy, the European Resuscitation Council (ERC) introduced a separate chapter about post-resuscitation care in the 2015 guidelines [3]. One of the key elements to improve survival rate after sudden cardiac arrest may be the enhancement of post-resuscitation therapy.

The post-cardiac arrest brain injury remains the main cause of mortality in the post-cardiac arrest period, being as high as 68% after OHCA and 25% after IHCA [4]. These data show that one of our leading goals during post-resuscitation therapy is to prevent secondary brain damage and guide a proper neuroprotective therapy.

We are going to point out the importance and process of recent neuroprotective strategies in this chapter. The role of normoxia, normocapnia, normoglycemia, seizure control, sedation and pharmacotherapy will be discussed in brief and we will work out in more details the place of control of hemodynamic parameters and targeted temperature management (TTM) in post-cardiac arrest condition.

2. Post-cardiac arrest syndrome

The post-resuscitation disease, later called post-cardiac arrest syndrome (PCAS) was first described in 1972 by Vladimir Negovsky as the unnatural pathophysiological state created by successful cardiopulmonary resuscitation (CPR) once resumption of spontaneous circulation has been achieved after whole body ischemia [5].

Post-cardiac arrest syndrome is the unique and complex combination of pathophysiological processes, including post-cardiac arrest brain injury, post-cardiac arrest myocardial dysfunction, systemic ischemia-reperfusion response and the unresolved pathological process causing cardiac arrest [6]. The contribution of each of these components in an individual patient depends on several factors including comorbidities, duration of the ischemic insult and the cause of cardiac arrest itself.

2.1. Systemic ischemia-reperfusion response

The pathophysiology of PCAS is very complex and contains processes that are still not completely understood. It is dominated by ischemia and reperfusion followed by systemic inflammatory response syndrome (SIRS). The reduced oxygen supply during ischemia or the so-called "no-flow phase" brings a decrease in adenosine-triphosphate synthesis and leads to cell membrane depolarization and opens the voltage-dependent calcium channels. Intracytoplasmic calcium level increases as a consequence that is responsible for cell damage. During reperfusion or the "low-flow phase", blood flow restores but oxygen radical species are formed. The hydroxyl radical is cytotoxic and causes cell death [7]. The plasma of patients after OHCA was analyzed and an acute pro-oxidant state within the cells was showed [8]. Cytokine production, activation of complements and expression of leukocyte adhesion molecules stimulate the activation of polymorphonuclear neutrophils and lead to systemic inflammation and multiorgan failure. Inflammatory response syndrome is associated with changes of hemostasis effecting secondary damage in endothelium that is followed by thrombus formation and increased capillary permeability [9]. It is important to point out that the worsening of visceral lesions occurs during reperfusion and is extended over the first hours, explaining the potential efficacy of delayed TTM. The clinical manifestation of PCAS-induced inflammatory response reaction shows a lot of similarities with sepsis [9]. The clinical picture is dominated by hemodynamic instability in the first hours and days. It leads to organ hypoperfusion if untreated and a consecutive multiorgan failure. The hypoperfusion of brain, caused by these hemodynamic changes, may lead to secondary brain damage and worse neurological outcome in this patient group.

2.2. Post-cardiac arrest brain injury

The anoxic-ischemic neurological damages remain the leading cause of death occurring in patients resuscitated from cardiac arrest [4]. Its clinical manifestation is very widespread: coma, seizures, myoclonus, varying degrees of neurocognitive dysfunction and brain death may occur [10].

The neurological damage is initiated during "no-flow phase", but is accelerated during the "low-flow period". The triggers of brain injury after cardiac arrest and a successful resuscitation are: excitotoxicity, disrupted calcium homeostasis, formation of free radicals, activation of protease cascades and apoptosis signaling pathways [11, 12]. Most of these pathways activate over hours to days after the return of spontaneous circulation (ROSC). If cardiac arrest is prolonged, failure of microcirculatory reperfusion may appear despite adequate cerebral perfusion pressure (CPP) leading to micro-infarctions. On the other hand, in the first minutes immediately after ROSC, a macroscopic hyperemia may occur that is caused by elevated CPP and impaired autoregulation [13]. As a consequence brain edema and reperfusion injury will exacerbate. Mullner et al. showed that a higher mean arterial pressure (MAP) did not improve the neurological outcome in the first 5 minutes after ROSC but if they were kept at a higher MAP in the first 2 hours after ROSC, the neurological outcome improved [14]. There are growing data to show that overload of oxygen during the initial phase after ROSC may be also harmful and can exacerbate cerebral damage through mitochondrial injury and free radical production [15].

Secondary brain injury may be evoked by a number of insults caused mainly by inappropriate post-cardiac arrest treatment in the first hours and days after cardiac arrest: hypo/hyperoxia, hypo/hypercapnia, hypotension, hypo/hyperglycemia, pyrexia, impaired cerebral autoregulation and brain edema.

One of the consequences of the primary brain damage is the impairment in cerebral autoregulation, however human data are limited [13]. It results that the cerebral perfusion varies with CPP in the acute and subacute phase of the disease. Experimental and clinical studies show that cerebral blood flow (CBF) and metabolic rate of cerebral oxygen consumption is decreased in the first 24–48 hours after ROSC due to increased cerebral vascular resistance [16].

Specific brain regions appear to be most commonly affected with events causing poor systemic circulation [17]. These regions are insulted because they lie in watershed vascular areas or their neurons are located at areas with a higher metabolic rate and oxygen/glucose demand more vulnerable to ischemia.

The neurological syndromes that occur in cardiac arrest survivors can be partially explained by the focal areas of brain injury [17]. The CA1 pyramidal neurons of the hippocampus are commonly damaged with prolonged ischemia, resulting impairment in memory functioning. Cerebellar Purkinje cell injury may result in ataxia, commonly manifesting as a gait disturbance from axial instability. Other commonly affected neurons include thalamic reticular neurons, the medium-sized striatal neurons and the pyramidal neurons in the layers 3, 5 and 6 of neocortex. With more prolonged periods of ischemia, arterial border zone regions can be appreciated macroscopically on neuroimaging. Patients with prolonged period of hypoxia followed by a global ischemic event appears to be susceptible to preferential injury to the subcortical white matter, in what appears to be a primary myelinolytic process. It is postulated that injury occurs preferentially in the subcortical matter in situations in which there is a significant period of alveolar hypoventilation, progressive acidosis and severe metabolic disturbances in the peri-arrest period.

2.3. Post-cardiac arrest myocardial dysfunction

Post-cardiac arrest myocardial dysfunction also contributes to the low survival rate after OHCA and IHCA [4]. However, this phenomenon is responsive to therapy and is reversible. Heart rate and blood pressure may be extremely variable immediately after ROSC caused by the transient increase in serum catecholamine concentration of endogenous and exogenous origin. When post-cardiac arrest myocardial dysfunction occurs, it can be detected within minutes of ROSC by appropriate monitoring. During the period with significant dysfunction, coronary blood flow is not reduced, indicating a true stunning phenomenon rather than permanent injury or infarction. This global dysfunction is transient and full recovery can occur, usually between 24 and 48 hours after the cardiac arrest. The responsiveness of post-cardiac arrest global myocardial dysfunction to inotropic drugs is well documented in animal studies [18]. In swines, dobutamine infusions dramatically improve systolic (left ventricular ejection fraction) and diastolic (isovolumetric relaxation of left ventricle) dysfunction after cardiac arrest [19].

2.4. Persistent precipitating pathology

The pathophysiology of post-cardiac arrest syndrome is commonly complicated by persisting acute pathology that caused or contributed to the cardiac arrest itself. On the other hand differential diagnosis and management of the precipitating pathology can be made more difficult by the symptoms and pathophysiologic changes caused by post-cardiac arrest syndrome. Some of the most frequent conditions leading to cardiac arrest are the followings: acute coronary syndrome, acute aortic syndromes, pulmonary embolism, pulmonary diseases (COPD, asthma bronchiale, pneumothorax), hypovolemia due to hemorrhage or dehydration, sepsis, central nervous system diseases and various toxidromes. The potential treatments are interventions specific for each disease guided by the patient's condition.

3. Tools of neuroprotection in post-resuscitation care

3.1. Normoxia and normocapnia

Arterial oxygen could be a modifiable component of patient care after cardiac arrest in order to deliver better neurological outcomes.

In the search for modifiable ROSC factors, the role of supplemental oxygen, which is often administered in high concentrations to patients after cardiac arrest, has come into controversy. Early oxygen administration can influence oxidative metabolism, respiratory markers, vasoconstrictive status and blood flow, and may thus be an important predictor of outcome [20]. Although it is intuitive that insufficient oxygen delivery can exacerbate cerebral anoxia, excessive oxygen delivery can also be harmful by increasing the amount of oxygen free radicals and subsequent reperfusion injury. Pure oxygen therapy after cardiac arrest has previously been shown to worsen neurological outcome in animal models and exposure to hypocapnia and hypercapnia after ROSC has been associated with poor neurological function at hospital discharge [20].

Oxygen creates a paradox when delivered to the damaged brain. If there is too little oxygen then potential anoxic injury may occur, while too much oxygen may increase the production of oxygen free radicals, leading to cellular injury and apoptosis [21].

In clinically relevant experimental models of cardiac arrest, hyperoxia has been shown to worsen the severity of oxidative stress, causing a greater loss of pyruvate dehydrogenase complex, impairment of oxidative energy metabolism and higher oxidation of brain lipids, culminating in more severe brain histopathologic changes and worse neurological deficits [21].

Kilgannon et al. reported data from adult intensive care units (ICU) of 120 US hospitals incorporated in a large administrative database named "Project IMPACT" and it included 6326 patients divided into three groups (hyperoxia, normoxia and hypoxia) according to the first partial pressure of oxygen in arterial blood (PaO_2) obtained within 24 hours following ICU arrival [22]. Arterial hyperoxia and hypoxia were defined as a PaO_2 higher than 300 mmHg and a PaO_2 lower than 60 mmHg, respectively. The authors found that in-hospital mortality was significantly higher in the hyperoxia group as compared with both the normoxia and the hypoxia group (63 vs. 45 and 57%, respectively).

In addition, among hospital survivors, patients with hyperoxia had a significantly lower likelihood of independent functional status at hospital discharge as compared with patients with normoxia (29 vs. 38%, respectively).

A secondary analysis showed a dose-dependent association between supranormal PaO_2 and risk of in-hospital death [23]. In particular, 25 mmHg increase in PaO_2 was associated with 6% increase in relative risk of death. Given that the median post-resuscitation PaO_2 in this sample was 231 mmHg, it appears that a high proportion of adult patients resuscitated from cardiac arrest have exposure to supranormal oxygen tension. Considering the linear increase in risk of death associated with PaO_2, these results suggest a need for clinical trials of a controlled oxygen therapy after resuscitation from cardiac arrest.

The ERC guidelines for post-resuscitation care recommend the avoidance of unnecessary arterial hyperoxia and a controlled reoxygenation strategy targeting an arterial oxygen saturation of 94–96% [3].

Carbon-dioxide (CO_2) may have neuroprotective properties, as it is thought that mild increase in its level improves cerebral perfusion and it has anticonvulsant, anti-inflammatory and antioxidants properties [24]. On the other hand, its decrease has been associated with neuronal injury in animal models and after traumatic brain injury.

Schneider et al. published an observational cohort study to observe the relationship between arterial CO_2 partial pressure ($PaCO_2$) and outcome in 16,542 patients admitted to the ICU after cardiac arrest [24]. This study was the first to report the relationship between $PaCO_2$ and mortality and an alternative marker of likely neurological outcome.

Within 24 hours of admission, about one in five patients had at least one episode of hypercapnia. Such abnormal values most often occurred within the first 2 hours of ICU admission and that hypercapnia may have been associated with non-ventricular fibrillation (VF) cardiac arrest and underlying respiratory disease. Compared with normocapnia, hypocapnia was associated with a greater risk of death and a lower likelihood of being discharged home among survivors.

On the other hand, hypercapnia was associated with similar mortality or outcome rates to normocapnia but with a higher chance of being discharged home among survivors.

Cerebral autoregulation is impaired after ROSC, but cerebrovascular reactivity to CO_2 is preserved. A decrease in $PaCO_2$ determines cerebral vasoconstriction with a consequent reduction of cerebral blood flow (CBF) whereas the opposite occurs when $PaCO_2$ is increased. There is evidence that CBF could be decreased in the post-resuscitation phase due to an imbalance between local vasodilators and vasoconstrictors but CO_2-mediated vasodilatation might reverse these abnormalities.

The ERC guidelines suggest adjusting ventilation to achieve normocapnia and monitoring the $ETCO_2$ (end tidal carbon dioxide level) and arterial blood gas values during post-resuscitation therapy [3].

3.2. Glucose control

Any stressful systemic injury, such as cardiac arrest, evokes a complex response involving glucoregulatory hormones such as catecholamines, glucagon and glucocorticoids. The increase of these hormones may result in glucose intolerance and hyperglycemia, as they can mobilize glucose and other energy substrates from storage pools. Glucose metabolism via anaerobic glycolysis is the only brain energy pathway that can sustain energy metabolism for any significant period of time (minutes) during an ischemic episode.

Unfortunately, it is common following CPR that the transport of glucose to brain tissues may become inadequate to satisfy cerebral metabolism [25]. Consequently, when cerebral perfusion is compromised, moderate hyperglycemia may facilitate glucose transport through the elevated blood glucose diffusion gradient that maximizes cellular glucose uptake.

On one hand, there are various studies that have shown that high blood glucose levels after ROSC are associated with increased mortality and poor neurological outcome for patients who experience OHCA. For IHCA patients, Beiser et al. reported that for patients without diabetes mellitus, both hypoglycemia and hyperglycemia were associated with decreased survival odds. However, for patients with diabetes mellitus, there was little association between blood glucose level and survival, except with extreme hyperglycemia [26].

On the other hand, there are several studies that have found out that normalization of blood glucose levels in critically ill patients with brain injury may be associated with greater risk of critical reductions in brain glucose levels and energy crises [27]. Therefore, acute stress hyperglycemia noted during the early post-ROSC phase might be a physiologic, rather than a pathologic response and attempts at interfering with this complex adaptive response may be harmful rather than protective.

It is proven that hypoglycemia needs to be avoided in critically ill patients. In a study by Arabi et al., mortality in patients with hypoglycemia was multipled compared to patients with conventional therapy [28]. Unrecognized episodes of hypoglycaemia are more harmful than the benefit of strict normoglycemia, especially in patients with brain damage [29].

The American Heart Association (AHA) guidelines do not recommend a target blood glucose range for post-ROSC patients [30]. The ERC guidelines suggest that blood glucose level should be maintained below 180 mg/dl (10 mmol/L) in these patients and that hypoglycemia should be strictly avoided [3].

3.3. Seizures control

Many of patients who remain comatose after successful resuscitation, will suffer from seizures. The appearance of seizures may be variable, from single focal onset through myoclonus to generalized tonic-clonic fit.

Acute post hypoxic myoclonus (PHM) occurs in about 18–25% of these patients, typically within the first 24 hours after CPR [31]. Commonly, the myoclonus appears days or weeks after the hypoxic episode when consciousness is regained. Myoclonus is a hyperkinetic movement disorder characterized as a sudden, jerky, shock-like movement. It can involve different body parts individually (focal), contiguously (segmental) or asynchronously (multifocal). When repetitive, the jerks may be regular or irregular, sometimes mimicking tremor.

There are several EEG findings in acute PHM: burst suppression (56%), spike-wave activity (37%), myoclonic status epilepticus (31%), diffuse slow background and waves (21%) and alpha coma (7%). These severe diffuse EEG abnormalities are consistent with marked diffuse cerebral dysfunction.

The exact neuronal damage and pathophysiology that gives origin to acute PHM is not clear. [32] Treatment is indeed challenging and no published guidelines exist as the hypoxic injury may lead to mixed and varying clinical findings of this myoclonus. Moreover, a drug treatment for one type may not work well in another or may even induce worsening [33].

3.4. Sedation

Sedative agents play a vital role in the management of patients with an acute brain damage. However, there is no evidence to support the defined duration of sedation neither the agent that should be used after cardiac arrest. Sedation acts to protect the brain against the extension of primary acute brain injury and secondary cerebral insults [34]. It has always been used in association with cooling methods, since the first non-randomized trials investigating targeted temperature management or therapeutic hypothermia (TH) effects on outcome. In this setting sedatives were often co-administered with muscle relaxants.

The main goals to use sedation during targeted temperature management are the reduction of oxygen consumption, control of shivering, the reduction of agitation and ventilator dyssynchrony, which may be detrimental for neurological recovery [34]. Clinically detectable shivering can increase systemic metabolic rate with 24–160% above baseline resting energy expenditure and increase inflammatory markers. The use of neuromuscular blocking agents to avoid shivering is controversial and we think it should be the agent of an ultimate case because it may mask seizures and its prolonged use (more than 1 day) may lead to muscle weakness, prolonged ventilation and ICU stay.

There are no data about the influence of outcome of sedatives used after cardiac arrest. A combination of hypnotics and opioids is used in the most of cases [35]. Short-acting drugs are preferred, for example, remifentanil, alfentanil and propofol.

3.5. Pharmacologic strategies

There is still lack of proved pharmacological interventions providing neuroprotection for patients after successful resuscitation. However, there are some promising drugs that may have some beneficial effect on neurological recovery in this patient group. Most of these agents have been studied in experimental research and only a few clinical data are achievable.

Xenon is one of the most commonly investigated pharmacologic treatments in post-resuscitation therapy. Pre-clinical studies have shown that it can prevent the development of ischemic-reperfusion brain injury [36]. A randomized single blind trial investigated the cerebroprotective effect of xenon in 110 comatose patients after OHCA [37]. One half of patients received xenon combined with therapeutic hypothermia and the other half was treated only with hypothermic therapy. They did not find any difference in survival and neurologic outcome after 6 months but there was less white matter damage controlled with magnetic resonance imaging (MRI) in the xenon-treated group. On the basis of these findings the efficacy of xenon must be investigated in further clinical trials at this patient group. Also we need to point out its disadvantages: it is still quite expensive and its storage needs special circumstances.

The impact of early high-dose erythropoietin was also investigated in patients after OHCA in a single blind randomized trial but neither mortality, neither Cerebral Performance Category (CPC) scale improved after this treatment, only rate of thrombotic complications increased [38].

Rosuvastatin was shown to improve survival, myocardial function and neurologic recovery in a rat model after successful resuscitation [39]. A combination of three drugs (lovastatin, minocycline and lamotrigine) was also studied in a mouse model after brain ischemia provoked by artery carotid occlusion [40]. As a result a decreased neurological deficit was reached suggesting a potential beneficial effect of this treatment in post-cardiac arrest therapy.

One of the promising, easily achievable and affordable drugs that may have potential benefit in neuroprotection after cardiac arrest is thiamine. It is a type of B vitamins that is essential for the proper functioning of nervous system. It modulates the activity of pyruvate dehydrogenase that is a main enzyme in Krebs cycle. It has been shown that mitochondrial dysfunction and impaired aerobic metabolism may be a cause of cerebral damage after cardiac arrest [41]. This led to the idea to investigate the effect of thiamine in mice after successful resuscitation [42]. Mice treated with thiamine after cardiac arrest had a better 10-day survival and improved neurological outcome than control individuals. The histology also showed an ameliorated brain injury after thiamine treatment. The investigators also checked the activity of pyruvate dehydrogenase in human blood in patients after successful resuscitation and found that it was significantly lowered compared to control healthy volunteers. We think thiamine may be a pharmacological pathway in treating post-cardiac arrest brain injury but its clinical effect and proper dosage need to be investigated in clinical trials.

3.6. Targeted temperature management

3.6.1. Principles and guidelines

Two trials published by the New England Journal of Medicine in 2002, involving patients who remained unconscious after resuscitation from cardiac arrest, compared therapeutic hypothermia (32–34°C for 12–24 hours) with standard treatment [43, 44]. These trials showed a significant improvement in neurologic function and survival with therapeutic hypothermia. This treatment method was incorporated into the resuscitation guidelines in 2005. For more than a decade, mild-induced hypothermia (32–34°C) was the standard of care for patients remaining comatose after resuscitation from OHCA with an initial shockable rhythm, and this has been extrapolated to survivors with initially non-shockable rhythms and to patients with IHCA.

Traditionally, therapeutic hypothermia (TH) refers to deliberate reduction of the core body temperature to a range of 32–34°C in patients who do not regain consciousness after ROSC.

Since the 2015 ERC guidelines, term targeted temperature management (TTM) is suggested to use instead of therapeutic hypothermia and the new recommendation is to keep patients' core temperature between 32 and 36°C [3]. However, this expression is not always unique and many use phrase therapeutic hypothermia for goal temperature 32–34°C and term TTM for goal temperature 36°C.

There are still several unanswered questions regarding targeted temperature management after cardiac arrest. We still do not exactly know which patients benefit from lower and which from a higher level of temperature. Only the detrimental effect of fever is proven of the effects of temperature in post-cardiac arrest syndrome. Further questions are when exactly to start cooling and how long to keep cooling, which still need more clinical trials to be answered.

The 2016 guidelines of American Academy of Neurology (AAN) on reducing brain injury following cardiac arrest try to give a more precise direction how to handle temperature management in this patient group [45].

Because patients with initial rhythm of ventricular fibrillation/ventricular tachycardia (VF/VT) or pulseless electrical activity (PEA)/asystole differ in causes of cardiac arrest and outcome, the guideline deals separately with these patient groups. It recommends the use of therapeutic hypothermia (32–34°C for 24 hours) if the initial rhythm was VF/VT and patients remain comatose after successful resuscitation. It also says that for patients with an initial rhythm of VF/VT or PEA/asystole TTM (36°C for 24 hours followed by 8 hours of rewarming to 37°C and temperature maintenance below 37.5°C until 72 hours) is likely as effective as TH and may be a good alternative. If the initial rhythm is PEA/asystole, than the use of TH possibly improves outcome over non-hypothermia treatment.

In 2013 a trial to investigate the benefits and harms of two targeted temperature regimens was conducted, called the Targeted Temperature Management (TTM) trial [46].

In the TTM trial, 950 all-rhythm OHCA patients from 36 ICUs in Europe and Australia were randomized for 36 hours of temperature control (comprising 28 hours at the target temperature followed by slow rewarm) at either 33°C or 36°C. Temperature was managed with intravascular or surface cooling devices for 36 hours, while the patients were sedated and mechanically ventilated. TTM at 33°C was associated with decreased heart rate, elevated serum lactate level, the need for increased vasopressor support and a higher extended cardiovascular SOFA score compared with TTM at 36°C. However, it is important to point out the higher proportion of bystander witnessed cardiac arrest (90%) and of bystander CPR (73%). Moreover, the time to start basic life support (BLS) was shorter in both groups, among 1 minute. These facts by themselves would provide an improvement in the outcome of patients regardless the hypothermia. Nevertheless, the median time of ROSC was 25 minutes in both groups.

The TTM trial has also been criticized because the temperature was tightly controlled and it took a short time to reach 33°C, but also because the whole trial cohort was less ill than in previous trials. It should be taken into account that the previous studies were performed several years ago, and that during the last decade the intensive care therapy has improved a lot itself [47].

It is also a very important fact that in TTM trial there was no fever during the therapy. When comparing the TTM trial and the previous trial temperature results, we can appreciate that the temperature after re-warming was lower in the TTM trial [43, 44, 46].

Kaneko et al. conducted an observational study between January 2005 and March 2013 called the J-Pulse-Hypo Japanese prospective cohort. The objective of the study was to identify subgroups of patients who might be suitable candidates for lower targeted temperature during TTM after ROSC [48].

Participants were divided into lower (32–33.5°C) or moderate (34–35°C) temperature groups. In this study a favorable primary outcome was defined as CPC (Cerebral Performance Category) 1–2 on day 30. The subgroups of patients were divided and analyzed in the following way: age ≤60 vs. >60 years and resuscitation interval of ≤30 vs. >30 minutes.

The results demonstrated that the lower temperature group significantly improved the proportion of patients with favorable neurological outcomes in the subgroup of patients with a resuscitation interval of ≤30 minutes. There were some differences between this study and the TTM Trial, including shorter time to reach the targeted temperature (180 minutes), longer time at the targeted temperature (34 hours), and longer re-warming period (3 days).

When to start cooling is also an interesting and still unanswered question regarding TTM. It was shown in preclinical studies that initiating cooling as soon as possible after resuscitation improves neurologic outcome [49]. Clinical studies investigating the beneficial effects of cooling initiated in pre-hospital setting did not show positive outcome. A Cochrane review studied 7 trials (2369 patients) investigating the effect of pre-hospital cooling on survival, cerebral injury, side effects, quality of life and length of hospital stay [50]. There was no difference in survival between pre-hospital and intra-hospital cooling groups, neither in neurologic outcome. The rate of re-arrests was higher among patients who received pre-hospital cooling in four of the investigated trials.

The guidelines of AAN do not suggest the use of pre-hospital cooling while it is ineffective in improving neurological outcome and survival [45]. One of the explanations for this phenomenon may be the fact, which has been already mentioned, that there are some complex mechanisms leading to post-cardiac arrest brain injury appearing some hours after ROSC. On the other hand high volumes of cold infusions are used to initiate TTM during pre-hospital cooling leading to pulmonary edema and complications causing more harm than benefit. We also need to mention the heterogeneity of studied cooling methods in pre-hospital setting. To prove its efficacy or inefficiency further studies are needed.

3.6.2. *Beneficial effects in post-cardiac arrest syndrome*

Hypothermia provides significant cardiac and neurological protective effects through different pathways. Hypothermic mechanisms providing myocardial protection include improved energy production during ischemia, increased calcium sensitivity of myocytes, regulation of mitochondrial oxidative phosphorylation and preserved myocardial vascular autoregulation. All of these protective mechanisms would result in increased myocardial contractility.

After a post-anoxic injury, hypothermia may also protect cerebral function through decreasing apoptosis, reducing the release of excitatory (glutamate and dopamine) neurotransmitters, attenuating the reactive oxygen species production, preserving the blood-brain barrier, providing protection of cerebral microcirculation and decreasing intracranial pressure. Hypothermia decreases the cerebral metabolic rate of oxygen by about 6% for each 1°C reduction in core temperature and this may reduce the release of excitatory amino acids and free radicals.

Shivering will increase metabolic and heat production, thus reducing cooling rates. The occurrence of shivering in cardiac arrest survivors who undergo mild induced hypothermia is associated with a good neurological outcome. Occurrence of shivering was similar at a target temperature of 33 and 36°C.

Mild induced hypothermia increases systemic vascular resistance and causes arrhythmias (usually bradycardia). However, the bradycardia caused by mild induced hypothermia may be beneficial: it reduces diastolic dysfunction and its occurrence has been associated with good neurological outcome.

3.6.3. Side effects

Therapeutic hypothermia is an effective tool in neuroprotection after cardiac arrest, however it may cause several side effects that need to be monitored and declined during its use. Polyuria and electrolyte abnormalities such as hypophosphatemia, hypokalemia, hypomagnesemia and hypocalcemia may appear.

Insulin sensitivity and insulin secretion are decreased, that lead to hyperglycemia. Moreover, coagulation system can get impaired and bleeding risk is increased.

Hypothermia can impair immune system and extend infection rates. It is associated with an increased incidence of pneumonia, although the use of prophylactic antibiotics may prevent it to emerge.

The clearance of sedative drugs and neuromuscular blockers is reduced by up to 30% at a core temperature of 34°C. Clearance of sedative and other drugs will be closer to normal at a temperature of 37°C.

3.6.4. Practice of cooling

Whenever the indication is established the hypothermic treatment should be started as soon as possible. The trial performed in 2002 had the induction within 6–26 hours, with a median of 8 hours [43].

Hypothermic treatment and TTM has three phases such as induction of cooling, maintenance and rewarming.

Cooling may be delivered via external, internal and combined cooling methods. External cooling is carried out by traditional icepacks placed on the groin, axilla and sides of neck; surface temperature changer devices with thermo-feedback function such as blankets or self-adhesive plastic fluid-containers or cooling helmets over the head of the patient.

Internal cooling means intrabody cooling as intravascular, intrabladder or intragastrical method. It may be delivered via infusion of 30 ml/kg of 4°C saline, which decreases core temperature by 1.5°C. Intravascular cooling enables more precise control than external methods. The most precise temperature control with the fastest induction, reaction to temperature changes and rewarming is achievable via endovascular heat-exchange catheter. This latter is the most expensive method on the field.

3.6.5. Practice of TTM and post-cardiac arrest therapy in Semmelweis University Heart and Vascular Center

- Protocolisation: our cardiac ICU has a prospective protocol of care to anticipate, monitor, and treat each of the impaired organ functions by optimizing systemic perfusion, restoring metabolic homeostasis and support organ system function to increase the likelihood of survival with potentially good neurological outcome.
- Technical background: our cardiac ICU has 11 monitored beds, with central monitoring system as well. Seven invasive mechanical ventilators, two non-invasive mechanical ventilators

and four intraaortic balloon pumps are available. For patients who need mechanical circulatory support extracorporeal membrane oxygenator (ECMO)/ventricular assist device (VAD) background is available by the cardiac surgeons and cardiac surgical ICU.

- TTM target temperature: 33°C. The target time to achieve target temperature is usually 3–6 hours using thermo-feedback blanket device (**Figure 1**) and 1–2 hours using intravascular cooling catheters. Latter is rarely used due to the price of the catheter. The maintenance duration of target temperature is 24 hours. Rewarming duration is set to 0.25°C/hour that means approximately 16 hours. Invasive hemodynamic monitoring during TTM is also used but only upon the attending physician's preference and the equipment availability.
- Intubation and mechanical ventilation is always obligatory during TTM since sedation and if needed neuromuscular blockade is also used in these patients. Midazolam is the choice of sedation if the patient is hemodynamically unstable and propofol, if the patient is stable. Opioids are administered to decrease the cerebral metabolic rate additionally.
- Tight monitoring of invasive blood pressure, rhythm, ECG morphology, diuresis, core temperature and hemodynamic variables is obligatory.
- Prevention is also started at admission: the post-cardiac arrest patients with circulatory impairment are at higher risk of decubitus, stress ulcer and infections.
- Sampling from trachea, pharynx, nose, groins for cultures are done at admission and empiric intravenous antibiotic therapy is initiated. Infection risk is 7–17% by the literature, but no significant effect on mortality was shown.
- We plan to establish a continuous EEG monitoring during sedation and TTM but it is available only in limited fashion at the moment.

3.7. Cerebral perfusion

Patients with post-cardiac arrest syndrome experience on-going oxidant damage, profound systemic inflammation with vasodilation, myocardial stunning and adrenal axis suppression, which commonly result in major hemodynamic instability. Targeted temperature management with a lower core body temperature affects circulatory variables also negatively. As we previously mentioned the injured brain commonly has a dysfunctional autoregulation. This leads to the fact that blood pressure alterations in the post-cardiac arrest period may influence on-going cerebral injury and eventual neurologic outcome [51]. With disruption of normal cerebrovascular autoregulation, CBF may become directly related to cerebral perfusion pressure, which is dependent on MAP.

Hypotension may lead to persistent tissue hypoperfusion after ROSC, which may produce secondary cellular injury after the initial insult.

Kilgannon et al. studied the time-weighted average mean arterial pressure (TWA-MAP) for the first 6 hours after ROSC [51]. It was found that arterial hypotension was common while relatively fewer patients had an intrinsic hypertensive surge. It was determined that TWA-MAP was associated with neurologic outcome. This association appears to be driven by the strong association between hypotension and poor neurologic outcome, as opposed to an association

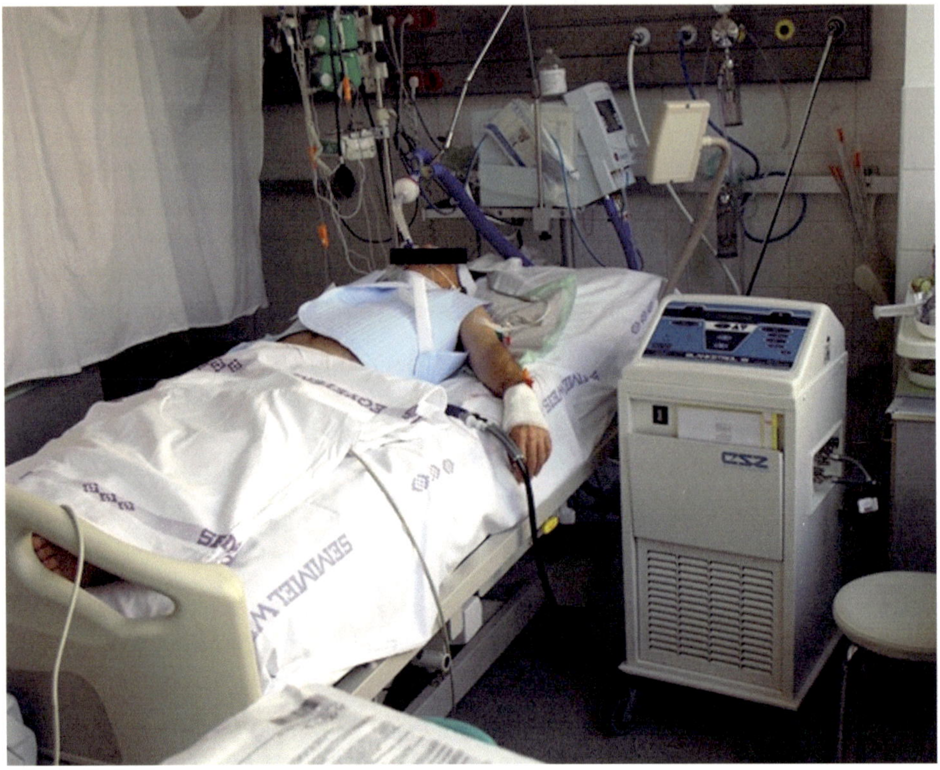

Figure 1. Thermo-feedback device used for external cooling in our practice.

between intrinsic hypertension and better neurologic outcome. In the analysis, there was a threshold effect with a TWA-MAP greater than 70 mmHg having the greatest association with good neurologic function, and they did not find higher MAP thresholds to be associated with favorable outcome.

The frequency and significance of post-ROSC arterial hypotension among cardiac arrest victims was measured at the time of ICU admission in a large, multicenter cohort study performed by Trzeciak et al. [52]. It was found that 47% of patients who survive cardiac arrest have post-ROSC hypotension, and two-thirds of these patients do not survive to hospital discharge. The presence of post-ROSC hypotension at the time of ICU admission is associated with an approximate two-fold risk of in-hospital mortality. It was identified that the post-ROSC condition is characterized by patchy microcirculatory cerebral hypoperfusion, and arterial pressure in the post-cardiac arrest period is a major determinant of the degree of cerebral perfusion impairment.

In spite of the studies that have tried to determine the appropriate blood pressure target after ROSC for a better neurological outcome, the results have not been conclusive. A recent study showed inverse effect between arterial pressure and survival [53]. In the absence of definitive data, the ERC guidelines recommend a target blood pressure that secures a satisfactory urine output (1 ml/kg/h) and a decreasing/normalizing lactate level taking into consideration the patient's normal blood pressure [3].

As a conclusion we can state that there are no clear data about the target blood pressure in post-cardiac arrest patients neither in shock patients [54]. There is lack of studies investigating the optimal target blood pressure in cardiogenic shock. However, it is showed that a target MAP of 65 mmHg may be satisfactory in septic shock patients, we need to point out that it is associated with a higher risk of acute kidney injury if the patient has a history of hypertension [55]. The main message of these findings is that the target blood pressure should be individualized to secure a proper perfusion of organs and an adequate perfusion of brain to prevent further secondary cerebral damage.

3.8. Hemodynamic monitoring during post-cardiac arrest syndrome and the hemodynamic effects of therapeutic hypothermia: a case control study (preliminary data)

We think that an expanded hemodynamic monitoring may be a more precise and useful tool to guide the hemodynamic management of post-cardiac arrest patients than observing only blood pressure. As we mentioned previously, there are several components leading to hemodynamic instability in this patient group and we need to mention also the complexity of the precipitating pathology causing cardiac arrest. To monitor cardiac output and its components (preload, afterload and contractility) gives a more synthetic picture about the condition of the patient's circulation and consecutive organ perfusion.

The most ideal method should be the least invasive providing the most information about the patient's circulatory condition with a simple usability. Echocardiography is a method that helps in characterizing the hemodynamic disorders, selecting the most optimal therapeutic intervention and assessing the response to it [54]. On the other hand it should be mentioned as a limitation that it is not a continuous technique for hemodynamic monitoring and it needs a lot of time of practice to reach an adequate level of usage.

Pulmonary artery catheter (PAC) provides important information about hemodynamic variables and tissue perfusion but it is one of the most invasive tools and there is no evidence about its superiority over other monitoring methods [56]. It is not the most useful system in determining preload because it measures only static parameters (central venous pressure and pulmonary occlusion pressure) instead of dynamic variables. The 2015 European Society of Intensive Care Medicine (ESICM) consensus on hemodynamic monitoring does not recommend its routine use in shock only in refractory shock with right ventricular dysfunction [54].

Transpulmonary thermodilution devices like PiCCO™ (Pulse index Contour Cardiac Output) are less invasive than PAC and they still provide enough precise information to be used in critically ill patients. Its additive advantage is the possibility to measure dynamic variables in fluid management. Tagami et al. validated this method in post-cardiac arrest patients even if therapeutic hypothermia (32–34°C) was used [57].

Recently developed non-invasive methods using pulse contour analysis and volume clamp technique to measure cardiac output should be limited to perioperative use because its value during shock, vasopressor therapy or targeted temperature management is questionable [54].

There is no evidence if the use of these methods affects patients' outcome in critical care not even in post-resuscitation therapy. Taking the above mentioned findings altogether we think

PiCCO™ monitoring system may be a suitable tool in post-cardiac arrest patients hemodynamic monitoring. There is still lack of evidence which hemodynamic variables should be monitored and which parameters should be targeted.

The aim of our study was to investigate if the use of PiCCO™ monitoring and the PiCCO™-guided hemodynamic assessment of post-cardiac arrest patients affect the survival, length of ventilation, length of ICU stay and the application of catecholamines. We also investigated the changes of hemodynamic variables during therapeutic hypothermia and were interested in how the most important tool of neuroprotection in post-cardiac arrest syndrome affects hemodynamics.

3.8.1. Patients and methods

We enrolled comatose patients after successful resuscitation who received therapeutic hypothermia and were treated in Semmelweis University Heart and Vascular Center between 2008 January and 2012 July. Inclusion and exclusion criteria are specified in **Figure 2**. We excluded patients who were given hypothermic therapy with physical cooling and ice packs, because the target temperature was not reached in most of the cases.

The post-resuscitation therapy and therapeutic hypothermia was initiated as soon as possible after the admission following the ERC guideline. The goal temperature was 32–34°C according to the even actual protocol (that is the reason we use term "therapeutic hypothermia" instead of "targeted temperature management"). The hypothermic treatment contained three phases: induction, maintenance and rewarming. The patients received 30 ml/kg cold (4°C) crystalloids in

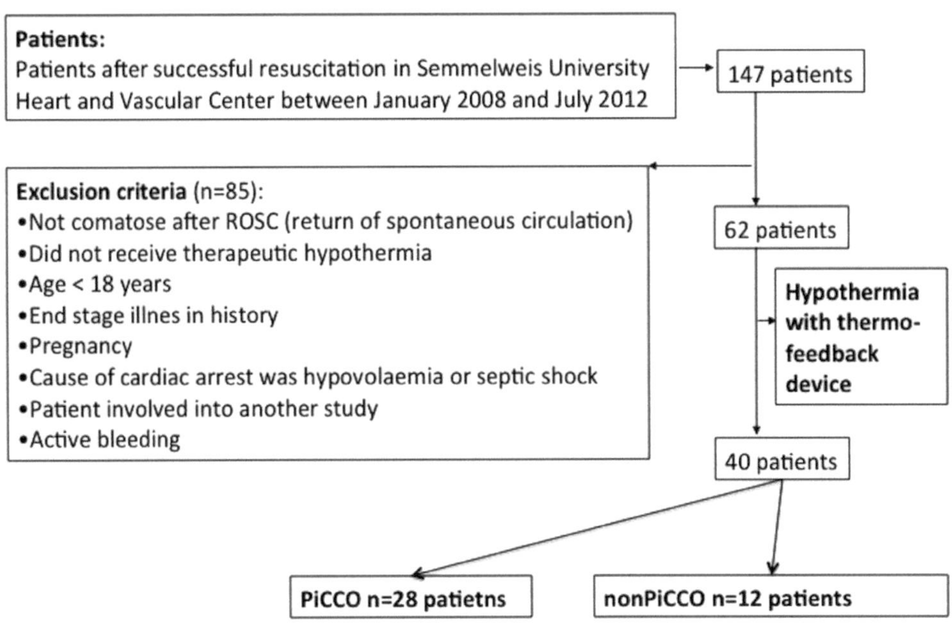

Figure 2. Inclusion and exclusion criteria.

the induction phase and were further cooled with Blanketrol III™ (Cincinatti SubZero) thermo-feedback device. The same device was used during the maintenance phase. The rewarming was a passive process where we tried to keep the 0.25°C/h rewarming speed. The patients' temperature was measured with an esophageal thermometer and they were sedated with benzodiazepine and opioids given intravenously. If it was indicated, we performed coronarography and percutanous coronary intervention before initiating hypothermia.

Patients were divided into two groups on the basis of what type of hemodynamic monitoring has been administered. We monitored by the members of nonPiCCO group oxygen saturation, ECG, invasive arterial blood pressure, central venous pressure, diuresis, blood gas parameters and serum lactate level. The patients' vasopressor, inotrope and fluid therapy was guided on the basis of these variables.

The previously mentioned monitoring and interventions were augmented with PiCCO™ (Pulsion Medical System) thermodilution device in PiCCO group. We accomplished a measurement at the initiation of hypothermia and performed it every 6 hours in the first 48 hours of treatment. The following variables were controlled: cardiac index (CI: $l/min/m^2$), systemic vascular resistance index (SVRI: dyn sec/cm^5), global end-diastolic volume index (GEDI: l/m^2), extravascular lung water index (ELWI: $ml/kg/m^2$).

The allocation of patients was directed by the access of the thermodilution device. Mortality, circumstances of CPR, length of ventilation and ICU stay and the usage of catecholamine therapy were recorded in both groups and compared. In PiCCO group, the hemodynamic variables (CI, SVRI, GEDI, ELWI) were controlled at the initiation of hypothermia, in the 12th, 24th and 48th hour of hypothermia and after rewarming. The statistical analysis was performed with two-tailed t-test and Mann-Whitney test when we compared the two groups. We used Wilcoxon test and Bonferroni correction in analyzing the PiCCO measurements. Significance of p value was set at <0.05. The Semmelweis University Regional and Institutional Committee of Science and Research Ethics accepted our study.

3.8.2. Results

We treated 147 successfully resuscitated patients in Semmelweis University Heart and Vascular Center between 2008 January and 2012 July. On the basis of our inclusion and exclusion criteria 40 patients were enrolled into our study: 28 in PiCCO group and 12 in nonPiCCO group. There was no significant difference in demographic data and the circumstances of CPR between the two groups (**Table 1**).

The survival (**Figure 3**), length of ventilation and length of ICU stay were also similar in both groups (**Table 1**). Length of ventilation was 5 ± 3 days in PiCCO and 6 ± 5 days in nonPiCCO group, respectively ($p = 0.57$). The patients in PiCCO group spent 7 ± 4 days at ICU and the members of nonPiCCO group 8 ± 5 days ($p = 1.00$).

In the usage of catecholamines we found that patients in nonPiCCO group received less vasopressors and inotropes than patients in PiCCO group (PiCCO: 71% of patients vs. nonPiCCO: 58% of patients), however the difference was not significant **(Table 2)**.

	PiCCO (n = 28)	nonPiCCO (n = 12)	p
Age (years)	62 ± 10	69 ± 8	**0.095**
Male	82%	67%	**0.25**
Female	18%	33%	
OHCA	64%	46%	**0.22**
IHCA	36%	54%	
Time until ROSC (minutes)	13 ± 6	17 ± 4	**0.059**
Initial rhythm			
VF/pnVT	63%	58%	**0.4**
PEA/Asy	37%	42%	
Bystander CPR			
Performed	72%	90%	**0.07**
Did not performed	18%	10%	
Length of mechanical ventilation (days)	7 ± 4	8 ± 5	**0.57**
Length of ICU stay (days)	5 ± 3	6 ± 5	**1**

OHCA: out-of-hospital cardiac arrest; IHCA: in-hospital cardiac arrest; ROSC: return of spontaneous circulation; VF: ventricular fibrillation; VT: ventricular tachycadria; PEA: pulseless electrical activity.

Table 1. The comparison of demographic data, circumstances of CPR, length of mechanical ventilation and length of ICU stay between PiCCO and nonPiCCO groups. Significance of p value was set at <0.05.

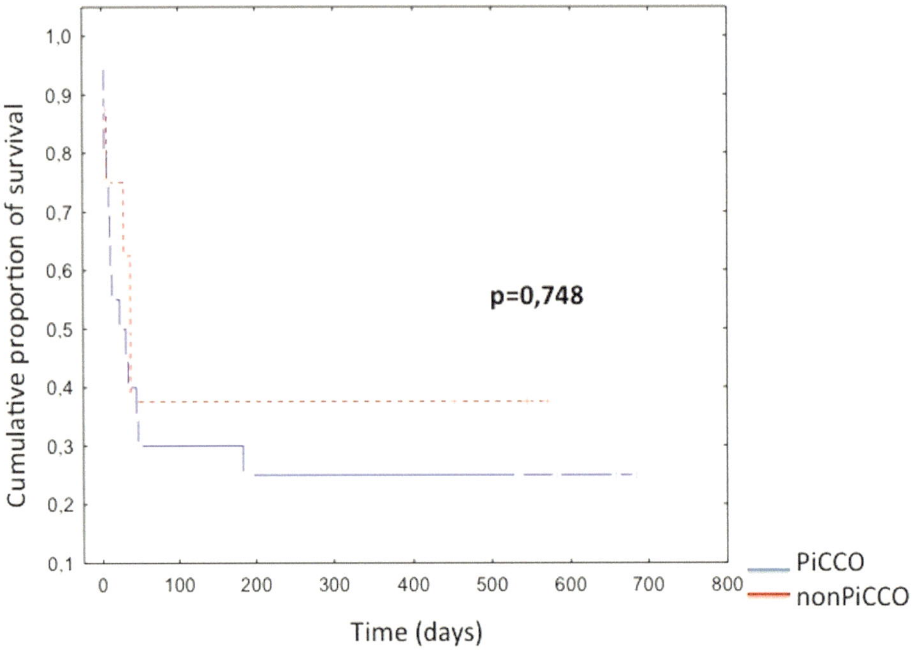

Figure 3. The comparison of survival between PiCCO and nonPiCCO group.

http://dx.doi.org/10.5772/intechopen.70593

Combination of catecholamines	PiCCO (n = 28) (%)	nonPiCCO (n = 12) (%)
0	29	42
1	36	25
2	21	8
3	14	25

Table 2. The comparison of catecholamine administration between PiCCO and nonPiCCO group.

In the course of the measurement of hemodynamic variables during therapeutic hypothermia there was significant difference in cardiac index and systemic vascular resistance index between the values in the 12th hour of hypothermia and after rewarming (CI: 1.8 ± 0.5 l/min/m^2 vs. 2.9 ± 0.9 l/min/m^2, $p < 0.001$; SVRI: 3686 ± 1264 dyn sec/cm^5 vs. 1627 ± 414 dyn sec/cm^5, $p < 0.001$) (**Figure 4**). Cardiac index decreased in the first 12–24 hours and showed improvement after this period. Systemic vascular resistance index changed parallel with cardiac index but the opposite way. The changes in ELWI and GEDI did not show significant difference during the examined interval.

3.8.3. Discussion

Post-resuscitation therapy as the fourth link of chain of survival is one of the mortality determining factors among post-cardiac arrest patients. One of the most important parts of

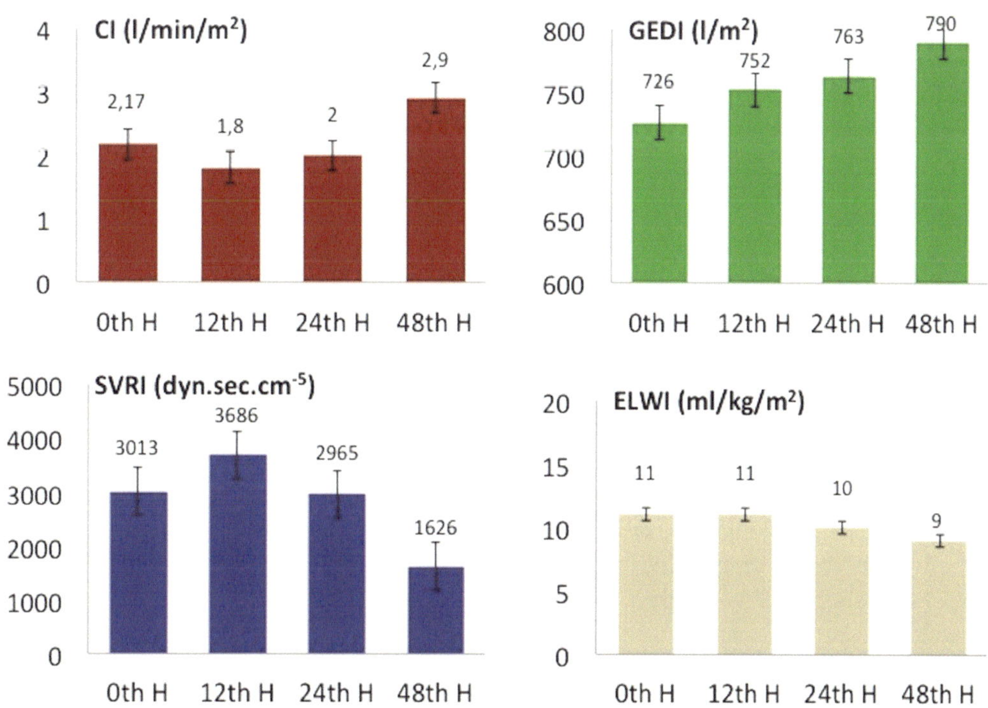

Figure 4. The changes of hemodynamic variables during therapeutic hypothermia (CI: cardiac index; SVRI: systemic vascular resistance index; GEDI: global end-diastolic volume index; ELWI: extravascular lung water index; H: hour).

post-resuscitation therapy is the proper attendance of cardiovascular disorders and an adequate guidance of hemodynamic management. The main goal is to secure a satisfactory organ perfusion and to prevent secondary brain damage by providing a sufficient cerebral blood flow despite the impaired cerebral autoregulation.

As we mentioned previously, there are several components leading to hemodynamic instability in patients after successful resuscitation [6]. There is pronounced vasodilatation due to systemic inflammatory response syndrome (SIRS) following an ischemia-reperfusion episode. The precipitating pathology itself resulted that cardiac arrest is a cardiovascular disease in most of cases. Cardiac stunning may develop after ROSC as a consequence of SIRS.

Targeted temperature management and therapeutic hypothermia may also affect hemodynamic variables of post-cardiac arrest patients in a negative manner: bradycardia, decrease in cardiac output and increase in systemic vascular resistance can evolve [58, 59]. As a consequence of lower temperature primarily during induction phase polyuria may occur resulting in hypovolemia [60]. Systolic and diastolic dysfunction was provoked in pigs while they were treated with hypothermia [61]. On the other hand these effects may be advantageous in this patient group because it has been shown that post-cardiac arrest patients with bradycardia had better outcome than patients whose heart rate was higher [62]. The increase of systemic vascular resistance is also a beneficial effect and may compensate the vasodilatory consequence of SIRS.

Bernard et al. used PAC as a hemodynamic monitoring in post-cardiac arrest patients and found that cardiac index was in tendency lower and systemic vascular resistance index was significantly higher in hypothermic group compared to normothermic patients [44]. It was also shown that cardiac index was in 66% of patients below 1.5 $l/min/m^2$ in the first 12 hours after ROSC in OHCA patients who were treated with therapeutic hypothermia. [63] They also used PAC to monitor hemodynamic variables.

As we mentioned it previously, we chose PiCCO™ monitoring system because it is less invasive than PAC and it was earlier validated in PCAS and therapeutic hypothermia [57]. We found during our measurements that cardiac index had the lowest value in the 12th hour of hypothermic treatment and it was significantly higher after rewarming. Investigating peripheral vascular resistance we measured the highest value of SVRI in the 12th hour of therapeutic hypothermia and a significantly lower value after rewarming. Our findings are similar to the measurements that have been performed with PAC.

On the basis of our results we think that there is a deteriorating hemodynamic instability during the first 24 hours after ROSC as a part of post-resuscitation syndrome. We also need to point out that treatment with lower temperature may also affect hemodynamic parameters. Our opinion is that taking these facts into consideration it is important to use a higher level of hemodynamic monitoring in this patient group to guide our hemodynamic therapy mainly if the patients are treated with targeted temperature management.

It is a different question if hemodynamic monitoring affects patients' outcome and mortality. There is no evidence which non-invasive, semi-invasive or invasive tool for hemodynamic monitoring should be used in critically ill patients. We think the answer is not simple and depends on patient, disease, patient's condition and the staff's practical knowledge. There is no evidence neither which parameters should we monitor and target during our therapy. To get closer to the answer more studies and randomized controlled trials are needed.

We were investigating in our study weather PiCCO™-guided therapy affects outcome in patients after successful resuscitation. There was no significant difference in demographic data and the circumstances of CPR between the two groups, so they were comparable. There was no difference in mortality, neither in the length of ventilation nor ICU stay between the groups. We found the same what was previously published in international literature. We found that in tendency more vasopressors and inotropes were used during the PiCCO™-guided therapy. It is very important to use these agents for the shortest time and in the lowest dose as possible to avoid side effects. PiCCO™-guided therapy, as it is shown in our study, may be a helpful equipment to fulfill this role.

The limitation of our study is the low number of study participants. We are planning to expand the investigation and we hope that with the increased number of patients enrolled we are getting a clearer result.

3.8.4. Conclusion

As a conclusion of our study, we can say that PiCCO™-guided therapy did not improve mortality, length of ventilation and ICU stay among our post-cardiac arrest patients. On the other hand we need to point out that it may play a role in conducting the vasoactive and inotrope therapy more adequately in this patient group. We proved that the decrease of cardiac index and increase of systemic vascular resistance index is observable also with PiCCO™ monitoring in the first 24 hours after successful resuscitation, during targeted temperature management.

4. Summary

A strong chain of survival can increase the chances of survival and recovery for victims of cardiac arrest. We summarized our recent knowledge about neuroprotective strategies after successful resuscitation in this chapter, that is, one of the most important parts of post-resuscitation therapy.

Normoxia, normocapnia, normoglycemia and a proper level of sedation must be maintained in order to avoid secondary brain damage. The use of pharmacologic strategies is questionable but thiamine may be a promising agent in improving neurological outcome. Its efficiency needs further clinical investigations.

Targeted temperature management is the most effective tool in our hand today. It has positive effect in the neurological recovery by decreasing fever, providing myocardial protection, slowing the brain metabolism and decreasing the inflammatory response. However, there are still many questionable topics in its implementation, like the targeted temperature, method, timing, duration of the therapy and the rewarming rate.

The proper management of hemodynamics in this patient group is also essential to secure a satisfactory brain perfusion, but the way of hemodynamic monitoring and the targets of hemodynamic variables are also subjects of further investigations. We think that PiCCO™-guided therapy can be a good direction to tailor vasopressor, inotrope and fluid therapy after cardiac arrest and during TTM.

Author details

Enikő Kovács[1†] and Endre Zima[2†*]

*Address all correspondence to: zima.endre@gmail.com

1 Department of Anesthesiology and Intensive Therapy, Semmelweis University, Budapest, Hungary

2 Heart and Vascular Center, Semmelweis University, Budapest, Hungary

†These authors are contributed equally.

References

[1] Berdowski J, Berg RA, Tijssen JG, Koster RW. Global incidences of out-of-hospital cardiac arrest and survival rates: Systematic review of 67 prospective studies. Resuscitation. 2010;**81**:1479-1487

[2] Perkins GD, Handley AJ, Koster RW, Castren M, Smyth MA, Olasveengen T, et al. European Resuscitation Council Guidelines for Resuscitation 2015 Section 2. Adult basic life support and automated external defibrillator. Resuscitation. 2015;**95**:81-99

[3] Nolan JP, Soar J, Cariou A, Cronberg T, Moulaert VRM, Deakin CD, et al. European Resuscitation Council and European Society of Intensive Care Medicine Guidelines for Post-Resuscitation Care 2015. Section 5 post-resuscitation care. Resuscitation. 2015;**95**:201-221

[4] Laver S, Farrow C, Turner D, Nolan J. Mode of death after admission to an intensive care unit following cardiac arrest. Intensive Care Medicine. 2004;**30**:2126-2128

[5] Negovsky VA. The second step in resuscitation—The treatment of the post-resuscitation disease. Resuscitation. 1972;**1**:1-7

[6] Nolan JP, Neumar RW, Adrie C, Aibiki M, Berg RA, Böttiger BW, et al. Post-cardiac arrest syndrome: Epidemiology, pathophysiology, treatment, and prognostication. A Scientific Statement from the International Liaison Committee on Resuscitation; the American Heart Association Emergency Cardiovascular Surgery and Anaesthesia; the Council on Cardiopulmonary, Perioperative, and Critical care; the Council on Clinical Cardiology; the Council on Stroke. Resuscitation. 2008;**79**:350-379

[7] Grace PA. Ischaemia-reperfusion injury. The British Journal of Surgery. 1994;**81**:637-647

[8] Huet O, Dupic L, Batteux F, Matar C, Conti M, Chereau C, et al. Potential role of hydroxyl radical-induced endothelial cell damage. Critical Care Medicine. 2011;**39**:1712-1720

[9] Adrie C, Adib-Conquy M, Laurent I, Monchi M, Vinsonneau C, Fitting C, et al. Successful cardiopulmonary resuscitation after cardiac arrest as a sepsis-like syndrome. Circulation. 2002;**106**:562-568

[10] Krumholz A, Stern BJ, Weiss HD. Outcome from coma after cardiopulmonary resuscitation: Relation to seizures and myoclonus. Neurology. 1988;**38**:401-405

[11] Bano D, Nicotera P. Ca^{2+} signals and neuronal death in brain ischemia. Stroke. 2007; **38**:674-676

[12] Pulsinelli WA. Selective neuronal vulnerability: Morphological and molecular characteristics. Progress in Brain Research. 1985;**63**:29-37

[13] Sundgreen C, Larsen FS, Herzog TM, Knudsen GM, Boegaard S, Aldershvile J. Autoregulation of cerebral blood flow in patients resuscitated from cardiac arrest. Stroke. 2001;**32**:128-132

[14] Mullner M, Sterz F, Binder M, Hellwagner K, Meron G, Herkner H, et al. Arterial blood pressure after human cardiac arrest and neurological recovery. Stroke. 1996;**27**:59-62

[15] Vereczki V, Martin E, Rosenthal RE, Hof PR, Hoffman GE, Fiskum G. Normoxic resuscitation after cardiac arrest protects against hippocampal oxidative stress, metabolic dysfunction, and neuronal death. Journal of Cerebral Blood Flow and Metabolism. 2006;**26**:821-835

[16] Beckstead JE, Tweed WA, Lee J, MacKeen WL. Cerebral blood flow and metabolism in man following cardiac arrest. Stroke. 1978;**9**:569-573

[17] Greer DM. Mechanisms of injury in hypoxic-ischemic encephalopathy: Implications to therapy. Seminars in Neurology. 2006;**26**:373-379

[18] Huang L, Weil MH, Tang W, Sun S, Wang J. Comparison between dobutamine and levosimendan for management of postresuscitation myocardial dysfunction. Critical Care Medicine. 2005;**33**:487-491

[19] Kern KB, Hilwig RW, Berg RA, Rhee KH, Sanders AB, Otto CW, et al. Postresuscitation left ventricular systolic and diastolic dysfunction. Treatment with dobutamine. Circulation. 1997;**95**:2610-2613

[20] Helmerhost HJF, Roos-Bloom MJ, van Westerloo DJ, Abu-Hanna A, de Kaizer NF, de Jonge E. Associations of arterial carbon dioxide and arterial oxygen concentrations with hospital mortality after resuscitation from cardiac arrest. Critical Care. 2015;**19**:348. DOI: 10.1186/s13054-015-1067-6

[21] Becker LB. New concepts in reactive oxygen species and cardiovascular reperfusion physiology. Cardiovascular Research. 2004;**61**:461-470

[22] Kilgannon JH, Jones AE, Shapiro NI, Angelos MG, Milcarek B, Hunter K, et al. Association between arterial hyperoxia following resuscitation from cardiac arrest and in-hospital mortality. JAMA. 2010;**303**(21):2165-2171. DOI: 10.1001/jama.2010.707.

[23] Kilgannon JH, Jones AE, Parrillo JE, Dellinger RP, Milcarek B, Hunter K, et al. Relationship between supranormal oxygen tension and outcome after resuscitation from cardiac arrest. Circulation. 2011;**123**:2717-2722. DOI: 10.1161/CIRCULATIONAHA.110.001016.

[24] Schneider AG, Eastwood GM, Bellomo R, Bailey M, Lipcsey M, Pilcher D, et al. Arterial carbon dioxide tension and outcome in patients admitted to the intensive care unit after cardiac arrest. Resuscitation. 2013;**84**:927-934. DOI: 10.1016/j.resuscitation.2013.02.014.

[25] Wang CH, Huang CH, Chang WT, Tsai MS, Yu PH, Wu YW, et al. Associations between blood glucose level and outcomes of adult in-hospital cardiac arrest: A retrospective cohort study. Cardiovascular Diabetology. 2016;**15**:118. DOI: 10.1186/s12933-0160445-y

[26] Beiser DG, Carr GE, Edelson DP, Peberdy MA, Vanden Hoek TL. Derangements in blood glucose following initial resuscitation from in-hospital cardiac arrest: A report from the national registry of cardiopulmonary resuscitation. Resuscitation. 2009;**80**:624-630. DOI: 10.1016/j.resuscitation.2009.02.011.

[27] Egi M, Bellomo R, Stachowski E, French CJ, Hart GK, Hegarty C, et al. Blood glucose concentration and outcome of critical illness: The impact of diabetes. Critical Care Medicine. 2008;**36**:2249-2255. DOI: 10.1097/CCM.0b013e318181039a.

[28] Arabi YM, Tamim HM, Rishu AH. Hypoglycemia with intensive insulin therapy in critically ill patients: Predisposing factors and association with mortality. Critical Care Medicine. 2009;**37**:2536-2544. DOI: 10.1097/CCM.0b013e3181a381ad.

[29] Losert H, Sterz F, Roine RO, Holzer M, Martens P, Cerchiari E, et al. Strict normoglycemic blood glucose levels in the therapeutic management of patients within 12 h after cardiac arrest might not be necessary. Resuscitation. 2008;**76**:214-220

[30] Callaway CW, Donnino MW, Fink EL, Geocadin RG, Golan E, Kern KB, et al. 2015 American Heart Association Guidelines Update for Cardiopulmonary Resuscitation and Emergency Cardiovascular Care. Part 8: Post-cardiac Arrest Care. Circulation. 2015;**132**:S465-S482. DOI: 10.1161/CIR.0000000000000262

[31] Bouwes A, Poppelen DV, Koelman JHTM, Kuiper MA, Zandstra DF, Weinstein HC, et al. Acute posthypoxic myoclonus after cardiopulmonary resuscitation. BMC Neurology. 2012;**12**:63. DOI: 10.1186/1471-2377-12-63.

[32] Crepeau AZ, Britton JW, Fugate JE, Rabinstein AA, Wijdicks EF. Electroencephalography in survivors of cardiac arrest: Comparing pre- and post-therapeutic hypothermia eras. Neurocritical Care. 2015;**22**:165-172. DOI: 10.1007/s12028-014-0018-4.

[33] Gupta HV, Caviness JN. Post-hypoxic myoclonus: Current concepts, neurophysiology, and treatment. Tremor and Other Hyperkinetic Movements. 2016;**6**:409

[34] Dell'Anna AM, Taccone FS, Halenarova K, Citerio G. Sedation after cardiac arrest and during therapeutic hypothermia. Minerva Anestesiologica. 2014;**80**:954-962

[35] Bjelland TW, Dale O, Kaisen K, Haugen BO, Lydersen S, Strand K, et al. Propofol and remifentanil versus midazolam and fentanyl for sedation during therapeutic hypothermia after cardiac arrest: A randomised trial. Intensive Care Medicine. 2012;**38**:959-967. DOI: 10.1007/s00134-012-2540-1.

[36] Wilhelm S, Ma D, Maze M, Franks NP. Effects of xenon in vitro and in vivo models of neuronal injury. Anesthesiology. 2002;**96**:1485-1491

[37] Laitio R, Hynninen M, Arola O, Virtanen S, Parkkola R, Saunavaara J, et al. Effect of inhaled xenon on cerebral white matter damage in comatose survivors of out-of-hospital cardiac arrest: A randomized clinical trial. JAMA. 2016;**315**:1120-1128. DOI: 10.1001/jama.2016.1933.

[38] Cariou A, Deye N, Vivien B, Richard O, Pichon N, Bourg A. Early high-dose erythropoietin therapy after out-of-hospital cardiac arrest: A multicentre, randomized controlled trial. Journal of the American College of Cardiology. 2016;**68**:40-49. DOI: 10.1016/j.jacc.2016.04.040.

[39] Qiu Y, Wu Y, Meng M, Luo M, Zhao H, Sun H, et al. Rosuvastatin improves myocardial and neurological outcomes after asphyxia cardiac arres and cardiopulmonary resuscitation in rats. Biomedicine & Pharmacotherapy. 2017;**87**:503-508. DOI: 10.1016/j.biopha.2017.01.007.

[40] Yu IC, Kuo PC, Yen JH, Paraiso HC, Curfman ET, Hong-Goka BC, et al. A combination of three repurposed drugs administered at reperfusion as a promising therapy for postischemic brain injury. Translational Stroke Research. 2017. DOI: 10.1007/s12975-017-0543-5 [Epub ahead of print]

[41] Bogaert Y, Sheu K, Hof P, et al. Neuronal subclass-selective loss of pyruvate-dehydrogenase immunoreactivity following canine cardiac arrest and resuscitation. Experimental Neurology. 2000;**161**:115-126

[42] Ikeda K, Liu X, Kida K, Marutani E, Hirai S, Sakaguchi M, et al. Thiamine as a neuroprotective agent after cardiac arrest. Resuscitation. 2016;**105**:138-144. DOI: 10.1016/j.reuscitation.2016.04.024.

[43] The Hypothermia after Cardiac Arrest Study Group: Mild therapeutic hypothermia to improve the neurologic outcome after cardiac arrest. The New England Journal of Medicine 2002;**346**:549-556.

[44] Bernard SA, Gray TW, Buist MD, Jones MB, Silvester W, Gutteridge G, et al. Treatment of comatose survivors of out-of-hospital cardiac arrest with induced hypothermia. The New England Journal of Medicine. 2002;**346**:557-563

[45] Geocadin RG, Wijdicks E, Armstrong MJ, Damian M, Mayer SA, Ornato JP, et al. Practice guideline summary: Reducing brain injury following cardiopulmonary resuscitation: Report of the Guideline Development, Dissemination, and Implementation Subcommittee of the American Academy of Neurology. Neurology. 2017;**88**:2141-2149. DOI: 10.1212/WNL.0000000000003966.

[46] Nielsen N, Wetterslev J, Cronberg T, Erlinge D, Gasche Y, Hassager C, et al. Targeted temperature management at 33°C versus 36°C after cardiac arrest. The New England Journal of Medicine. 2013;**369**:2197-2206. DOI: 10.1056/NEJMoa1310519.

[47] Nielsen N, Friberg H. Temperature management after cardiac arrest. Current Opinion in Critical Care. 2015;**21**:202-208. DOI: 10.1097/MCC.0000000000000203.

[48] Kaneko T, Kasaoka S, Nakahara T, Sawano H, Tahara Y, Hase M, et al. Effectiveness of lower target temperature therapeutic hypothermia in post-cardiac arrest syndrome patients with a resuscitation interval of ≤ 30 min. Journal of Intensive Care. 2015;**3**:28. DOI: 10.1186/s40560-015-0095-2.

[49] Jia X, Koenig MA, Shin HC, Zhen G, Pardo CA, Hanley DF, et al. Improving neurological outcomes post-cardiac arrest in a rat model: Immediate hypothermia and quantitative EEG monitoring. Resuscitation. 2008;**76**:431-442. DOI: 10.1016/j.resuscitation.2007.08.014.

[50] Arrich J, Holzer M, Havel C, Warenits AM, Herkner H. Pre-hospital versus in-hospital initiation of cooling for survival and neuroprotection after out-of-hospital cardiac arrest (review). The Cochrane Database of Systematic Reviews. 2016;(3): (Art No.: CD010570). DOI: 10.1002/14651858.CD010570.pub2

[51] Kilgannon JH, Roberts BW, Jones AE, Mittal N, Cohen E, Mitchell J, et al. Arterial blood pressure and neurologic outcome after resuscitation from cardiac arrest. Critical Care Medicine. 2014;**42**:2083-2091. DOI: 10.1097/CCM.0000000000000406.

[52] Trzeciak S, Jones AE, Kilgannon JH, Milcarek B, Hunter K, Shapiro NI, et al. Significance of arterial hypotension after resuscitation from cardiac arrest. Critical Care Medicine. 2009;**37**:2895-2903

[53] Bro-Jeppesen J, Annborn M, Hassager C, Wise MP, Pelosi P, Nielsen N, et al. Hemodynamics and vasopressor support during targeted temperature management at 33 degrees C versus 36 degrees C after out-of-hospital cardiac arrest: A post hoc study of the target temperature management trial. Critical Care Medicine. 2015;**43**:318-327. DOI: 10.1097/CCM.0000000000000691.

[54] Cecconi M, Backer D, Antonelli M, Beale R, Bakker J, Hofer C, et al. Consensus on circulatory shock and hemodynamic monitoring. Task force of the European Society of Intensive Care Medicine. Intensive Care Medicine. 2014;**40**:1795-1815. DOI: 10.1007/s00134-014-3525-z.

[55] Rivers E, Nguyen B, Havstad S, Ressler J, Muzzin A, Knoblich B, et al. Early goal-directed therapy in the treatment of severe sepsis and septic shock. The New England Journal of Medicine. 2001;**345**:1369-1377

[56] Rajaram SS, Desai NK, Gajera M, Cavanaugh SK, Brampton W, Young D, et al. Pulmonary artery catheters for adult patients in intensive care (review). The Cochrane Database of Systematic Reviews. 2013;(Issue 2 Art No.: CD003408). DOI: 10.1002/14651858.CD003408

[57] Tagami T, Kushimoto S, Tosa R, Omura M, Hagiwara J, Hirama H, et al. The precision of PiCCO measurements in hypothermic post-cardiac arrest patients. Anaesthesia. 2012;**67**:236-243. DOI: 10.1111/j.1365-2044.2011.06981.x.

[58] Polderman KH, Herold I. Therapeutic hypothermia and controlled normothermia in the intensive care unit: Practical consideration, side effects and cooling methods. Critical Care Medicine. 2009;**37**:1101-1120. DOI: 10.1097/CCM.0b013e3181962ad5.

[59] Kovacs E, Jenei Z, Horvath A, Geller L, Szilagyi S, Kiraly A, et al. Physiologic effects of hypothermia. Orvosi Hetilap. 2011;**152**:171-181. DOI: 10.1556/OH.2011.29006

[60] Raper JD, Wang HE. Urine output changes during postcardiac arrest therapeutic hypothermia. Therapeutic Hypothermia and Temperature Management. 2013;**3**:173-177. DOI: 10.1089/ther.2013.0015.

[61] Espinoza A, Kerans V, Opdahl A, Skulstad H, Halvorsen PS, Bugge JF, et al. Effects of therapeutic hypothermia on left ventricular function assessed by ultrasound imaging. Journal of the American Society of Echocardiography. 2013;**26**:1353-1363. DOI: 10.1016/j.echo.2013.06.021.

[62] Staer Jansen H, Sunde K, Olasveengen TM, et al. Bradycardia during therapeutic hypothermia is associated with good neurologic outcome in comatose survivors of out-of-hospital cardiac arrest. Critical Care Medicine. 2014;**42**:2401-2408. DOI: 10.1097/CCM.0000000000000515.

[63] Oksanen T, Skrifvars M, Wilkman E, Tierala I, Pettila V, Varpula T. Postresuscitation hemodynamics during therapeutic hypothermia after out-of-hospital cardiac arrest with ventricular fibrillation: A retrospective study. Resuscitation. 2014;**85**:1018-1024. DOI: 10.1016/j.resuscitation.2014.04.026.